yoga for kids

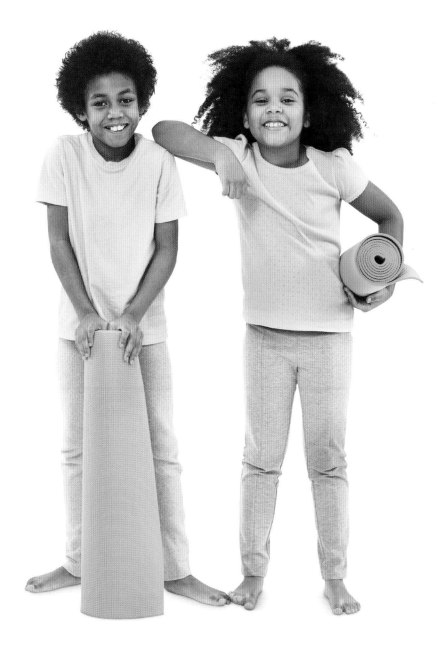

Written by **Susannah Hoffman**
Foreword by **Patricia Arquette**

Contents

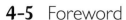

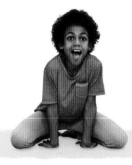

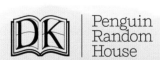

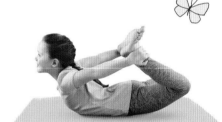

4-5   Foreword

6-7   Getting started

8-9   Om and Namaste

10-11   Shoulder stretches

12-13   Rocking the baby

14-15   Cat-cow stretch

16-17   Warm-up sequence

18-19   Downward dog

20-21   Hissing cobra

22-23   Bendy bow

24-25   Lion's breath

26-27   Resting child

28-29   Sailing boat

30-31   Energetic sequence

32-33   Mighty mountain

34-35   Low lunge

36-37   Mighty warrior

38-39   Invisible chair

DK Penguin Random House

Author Susannah Hoffman
Consultant Shari Vilchez-Blatt

Editor Katy Lennon
Senior Art Editor Fiona Macdonald
Senior Editor Lizzie Davey
Editorial Assistant Amina Youssef
Additional design Victoria Clark, Emma Hobson, Xiao Lin
US Senior Editor Shannon Beatty
US Editor Mindy Fichter
Jacket Coordinator Francesca Young
Jacket Designer Dheeraj Arora
Producer, Pre-Production Nadine King
Managing Editor Laura Gilbert
Managing Art Editor Diane Peyton Jones
Photographer Lol Johnson
Illustrator Kitty Glavin
DTP Designer Nityanand Kumar
Art Editor Seepiya Sahni

Creative Director Helen Senior
Publishing Director Sarah Larter

First American Edition, 2018
Published in the United States by DK Publishing
345 Hudson Street, New York, New York 10014

Text copyright © Susannah Hoffman, 2018
Foreword text copyright © Patricia Arquette, 2018
Copyright in the layouts and design of the Work shall be
vested in the Publishers.
DK, a Division of Penguin Random House LLC
18 19 20 21 22 10 9 8 7 6 5 4 3 2 1
001–310301–Sep/2018

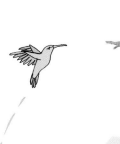
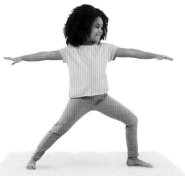
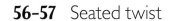

56-57 Seated twist

58-59 Cow face

40-41 Twisted eagle

60-61 Calming sequence

42-43 Stretching warrior

62-63 Little bridge

44-45 Confidence sequence

64-65 Half shoulder stand

46-47 Tall tree

66-67 Restful relaxation

48-49 Standing forward bend

68-69 Parts of the body

50-51 Happy baby

70-71 Glossary

52-53 Humming bee breath

72 Index

54-55 Monkey squat

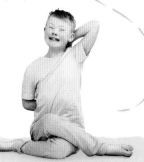
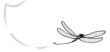

Published in Great Britain
by Dorling Kindersley Limited

A catalog record for this book
is available from the Library of Congress.
ISBN 978-1-4654-7541-1

DK books are available at special discounts when
purchased in bulk for sales promotions, premiums,
fund-raising, or educational use. For details, contact:
DK Publishing Special Markets, 345 Hudson Street,
New York, New York 10014
SpecialSales@dk.com

Printed and bound in China

A WORLD OF IDEAS:
SEE ALL THERE IS TO KNOW

www.dk.com

Safety information

Any physical activity has some risk of injury. Please be aware of your child's limitations and encourage them not to force or strain their bodies. Supervise and help your child as necessary. While the poses are helpful, they are not a substitute for medical advice or intervention if your child suffers from any medical condition.

Foreword

We live in a world of chaos, where doing everything at once is still not enough. There are seldom moments to stop, but we are only human. Like all people, I have run up against the wall more than once as a mother, an actor, and a human, moving through the changes that life deals you. Life waits for no one, so it is important to learn ways to survive, heal, and combat the fast world we live in. There is one thing that every doctor I have ever met has advised me when I am completely run down: "Do yoga!"

Children sadly are not immune to life's stresses and encounter them almost daily. Encouraging them to practice yoga from an early age allows them to find time to connect with their minds and bodies. This book is a great place to start!

Susannah Hoffman has taught yoga under the stars of the Sinai Desert in Egypt, next to inlets where wild dolphins swim, and in tents with drums beating. She has taught in London with cool, hard wooden floors under her feet, and has taught everyone from expectant mothers to movie stars. Now she has branched out into the world of publishing. With this wonderful book, Susannah aims to bring yoga into the homes and lives of children and their families.

Susannah has brought together her mindful nature as a mother and wisdom as a yoga teacher, making each page in this book simple, clear, and a joy to read. She instructs with an awareness of how best to help children deal with stress in their daily lives. A blessing for both kids and parents, she makes practicing yoga at home seem effortless!

Enjoy,

Patricia Arquette is a world-renowned actress who has won many awards, including an Oscar and a Golden Globe for her role in the film *Boyhood*. She has been a great believer in the powers of yoga and mindfulness since a young age.

Introduction

I was five years old when I started yoga and I have loved it ever since!
I hope this book inspires you in the same way.

Some of the poses in this book may feel difficult to do on some days
and easier on others. That's OK! We are all good at different things—
that's what makes us unique. Just know that you are doing it perfectly
for you on that day.

The poses have many benefits, such as lengthening and stretching your
body. Some bring courage and strength, while others are calming and good
for improving concentration. The breathing techniques allow us to become
still in our mind—to observe and let go of our fears and insecurities.

This book is designed to teach you how to listen to your body. Just choose
the poses or sequences that are right for you at that time.
Enjoy your yoga journey.

Namaste,

Susannah

Susannah Hoffman has been teaching yoga for more
than twenty years. She is a British Wheel of Yoga
Teacher and a senior teacher with Yoga Alliance
Professionals UK. She is one of the original teachers on
the Triyoga Teacher Training Diploma and created the
accredited "Teaching Yoga to Children" training.

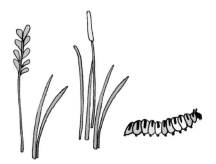

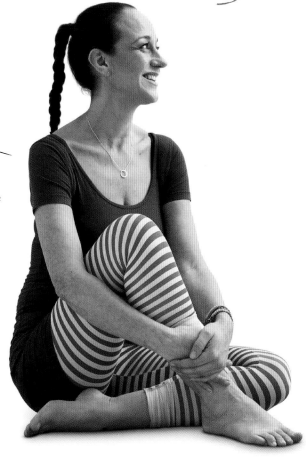

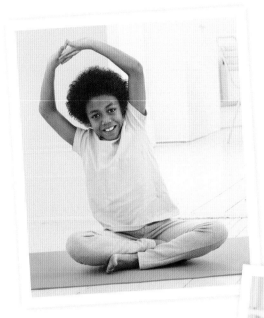

Getting started

Before you start practicing your poses, there are a few things that you need to know. These pages will tell you how to get the most out of this book.

Warming up

Pages 8–17 show the poses that you can do to warm up your body. Read and learn this section before moving onto the other poses.

Breathing

The way that you breathe when you are doing yoga is very important. Look out for tips on when to breathe in and out—they will help you get the most out of each pose.

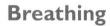

What you need

When doing yoga, wear comfy clothes that are easy to move in. Use a yoga mat to stop you from slipping. Yoga is best done with bare feet.

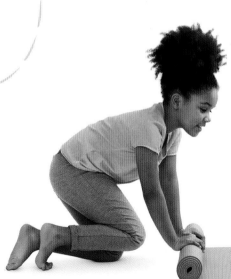

Using the book

The pose spreads teach you how to do the yoga moves safely, then the sequence pages link them together. Other pages focus on mindfulness.

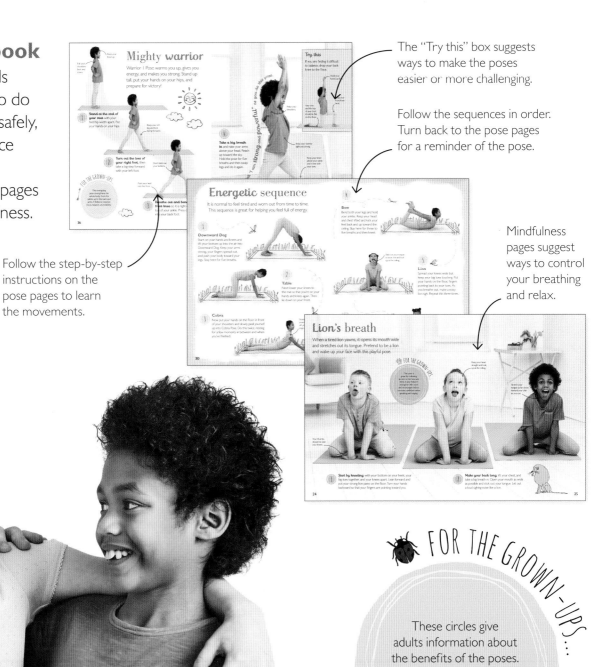

The "Try this" box suggests ways to make the poses easier or more challenging.

Follow the sequences in order. Turn back to the pose pages for a reminder of the pose.

Mindfulness pages suggest ways to control your breathing and relax.

Follow the step-by-step instructions on the pose pages to learn the movements.

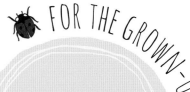

FOR THE GROWN-UPS...

These circles give adults information about the benefits of the poses. They also offer tips on how to encourage and help children learn each pose.

Yoga is for everybody!

Don't worry if you find some of the poses difficult—everyone is good at different things. Yoga takes practice, so just do what feels right for you.

Om and Namaste

Start your yoga journey by finding a space where you feel calm. Focus on yourself, relax, and think about your breathing. When you are finished, bring your hands together into Namaste position.

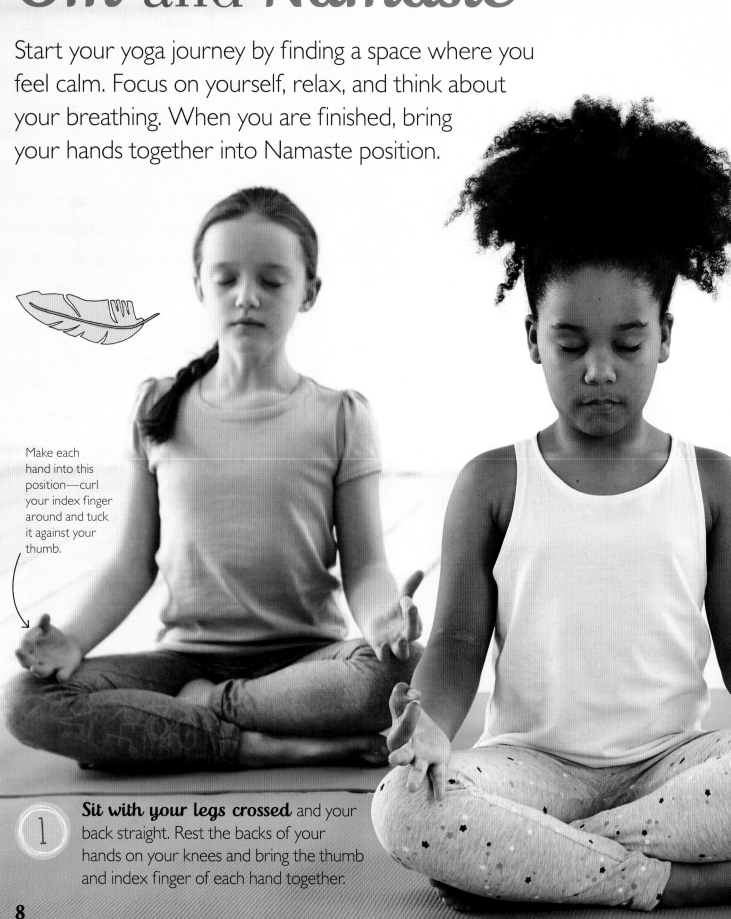

Make each hand into this position—curl your index finger around and tuck it against your thumb.

1 **Sit with your legs crossed** and your back straight. Rest the backs of your hands on your knees and bring the thumb and index finger of each hand together.

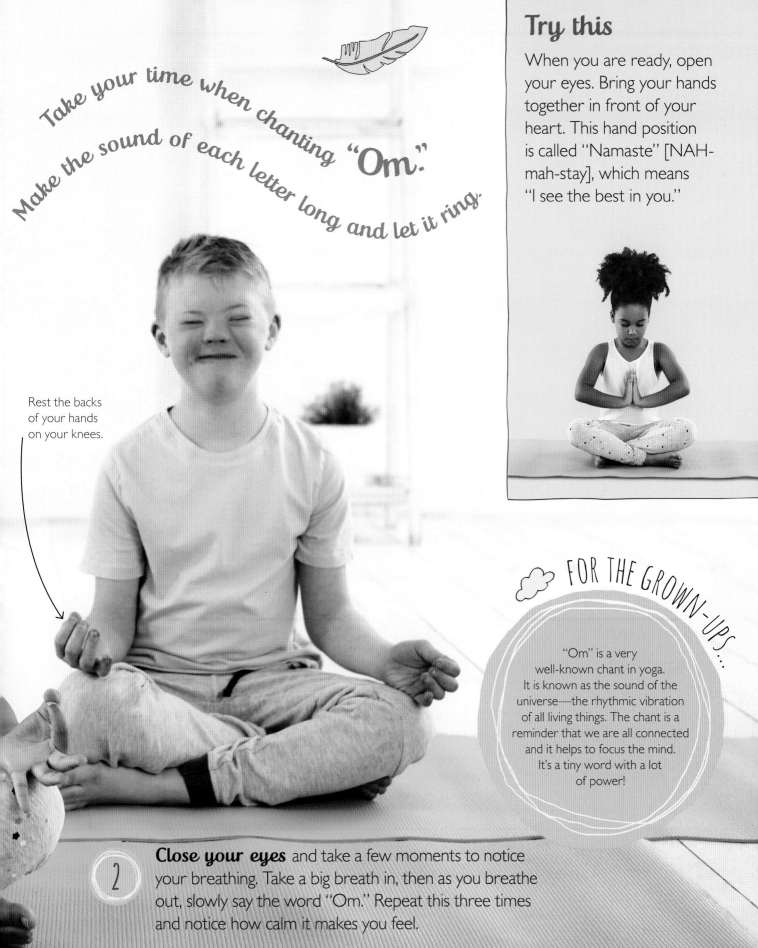

Take your time when chanting "Om."
Make the sound of each letter long and let it ring.

Rest the backs of your hands on your knees.

Try this

When you are ready, open your eyes. Bring your hands together in front of your heart. This hand position is called "Namaste" [NAH-mah-stay], which means "I see the best in you."

FOR THE GROWN-UPS...

"Om" is a very well-known chant in yoga. It is known as the sound of the universe—the rhythmic vibration of all living things. The chant is a reminder that we are all connected and it helps to focus the mind. It's a tiny word with a lot of power!

2 **Close your eyes** and take a few moments to notice your breathing. Take a big breath in, then as you breathe out, slowly say the word "Om." Repeat this three times and notice how calm it makes you feel.

Shoulder stretches

Shoulders can get very stiff, especially if you're carrying a heavy schoolbag around. These exercises are the best way to keep your shoulders relaxed.

Shoulder shrugs

These up-and-down shrugging movements help to get rid of any tightness in your shoulders.

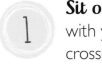

1 **Sit on the floor** with your legs crossed. Bring your shoulders up toward your ears.

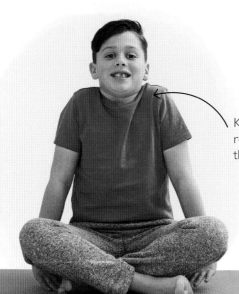

Keep your shoulders relaxed as you lift them up.

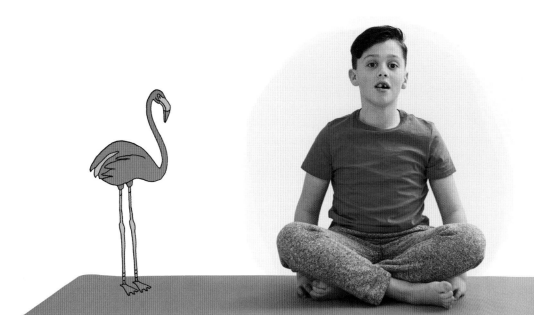

2 **Now, with a big sigh,** let your shoulders drop down again. Repeat steps 1 and 2 three times.

Seated side stretch

This move will stretch out your shoulders and the sides of your body at the same time.

Hold your arms straight out in front of you and link all of your fingers together.

Turn your hands out so that the backs of your fingers are facing you, then stretch your arms up above your head.

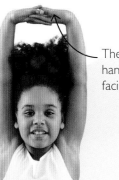

The palms of your hands should be facing the ceiling.

Take a big breath in and stretch up. As you breathe out, stretch to the side. Come back to the middle when you breathe in again, then breathe out and stretch to the other side.

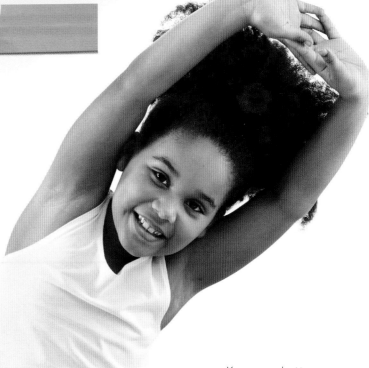

Keep your bottom on the floor and don't lean too far over.

Rocking the baby

Imagine that you are gently rocking a baby to sleep. What movement would you make? Try it out, with your leg playing the baby. This pose will help warm up your hips.

☆ FOR THE GROWN-UPS...

When children have growth spurts, it can take a while for their muscles to catch up with their bones. This means they often can have tight muscles. This pose will help stretch out tight hamstrings.

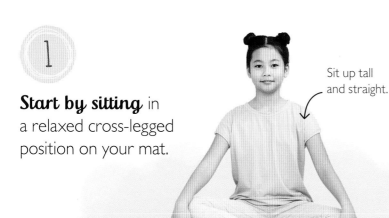

1

Start by sitting in a relaxed cross-legged position on your mat.

Sit up tall and straight.

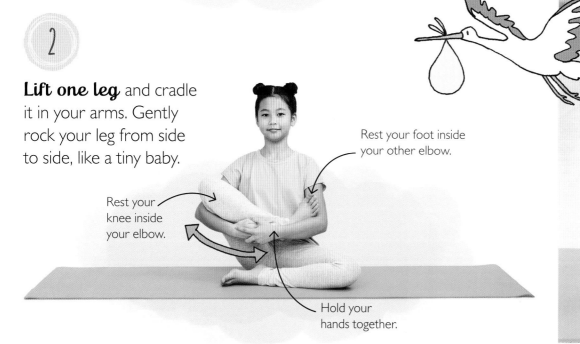

2

Lift one leg and cradle it in your arms. Gently rock your leg from side to side, like a tiny baby.

Rest your foot inside your other elbow.

Rest your knee inside your elbow.

Hold your hands together.

Try this

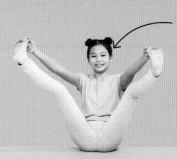

Keep this leg straight.

Keep your head and chest lifted up.

If it's hard to sit with one leg bent, you can straighten it out in front of you instead.

If you're ready for a more difficult position, try stretching out both your legs at once. See if you can balance long enough to say your name!

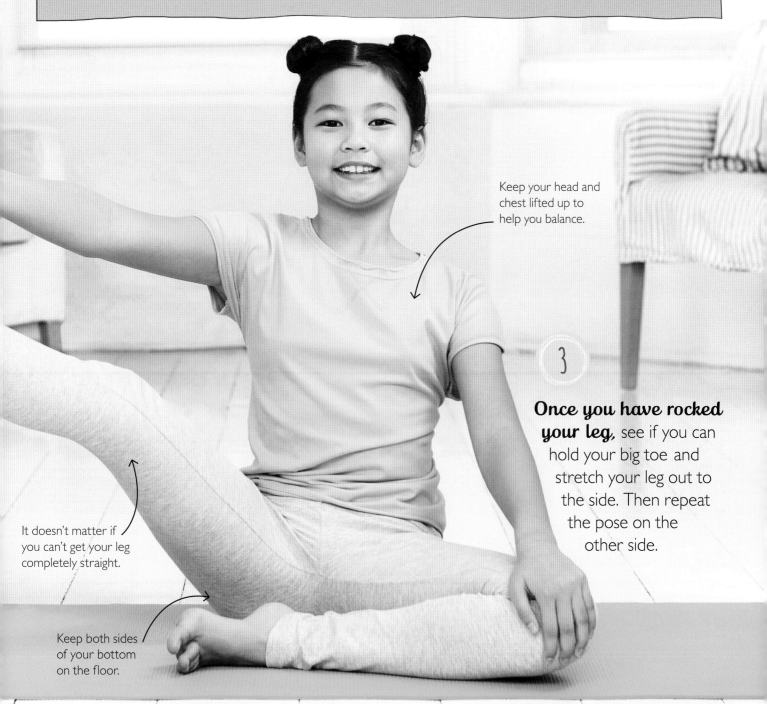

Keep your head and chest lifted up to help you balance.

It doesn't matter if you can't get your leg completely straight.

Keep both sides of your bottom on the floor.

3

Once you have rocked your leg, see if you can hold your big toe and stretch your leg out to the side. Then repeat the pose on the other side.

Cat-cow stretch

When a cat stretches, it round its back upward and when a cow moos it arches its back down. Cat-Cow Pose combines these two movements to help you stretch your back. You can even make animal noises as you do it!

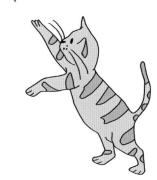

Kneel on your mat with your hands straight underneath your shoulders. Your knees should be directly under your hips. This is called Table Pose.

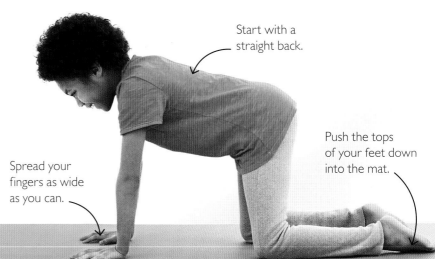

Start with a straight back.

Spread your fingers as wide as you can.

Push the tops of your feet down into the mat.

As you bend, imagine you are a COW standing in a field of daisies.

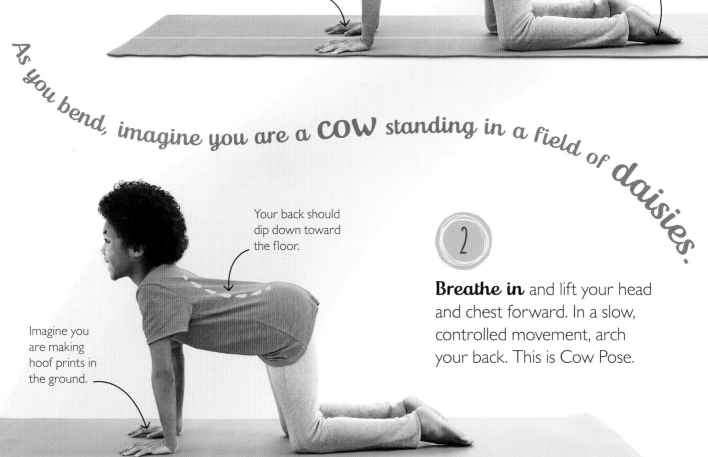

Your back should dip down toward the floor.

Imagine you are making hoof prints in the ground.

Breathe in and lift your head and chest forward. In a slow, controlled movement, arch your back. This is Cow Pose.

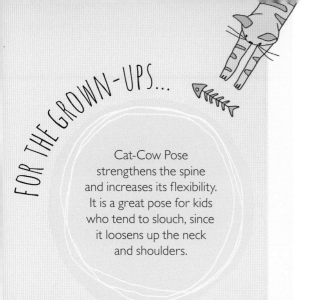
Try this

After you have practiced Cat-Cow Pose, try Tiger Pose. Start in the same position, but when you breathe in, lift up your leg like a tiger's tail.

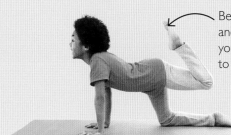

Bend your knee and try to bring your toes close to your head.

When you breathe out, swing your leg through your arms and try to touch your nose with your knee. Repeat these moves with the other leg.

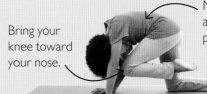

Make your back as rounded as possible.

Bring your knee toward your nose.

3

As you breathe out, arch your back and squeeze out all the air from your lungs. This is Cat Pose. Repeat steps 2 and 3 five times to completely wake up your spine.

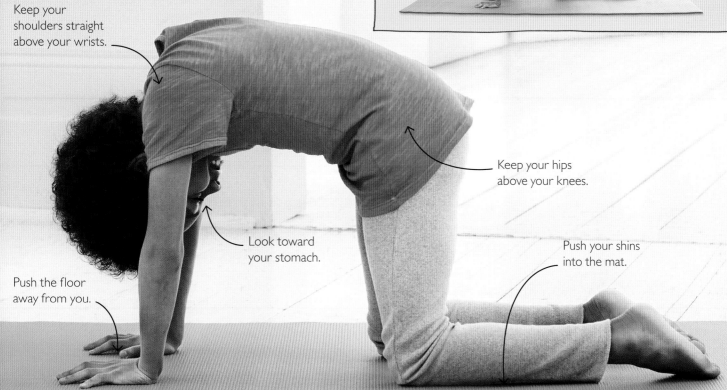

Keep your shoulders straight above your wrists.

Look toward your stomach.

Push the floor away from you.

Keep your hips above your knees.

Push your shins into the mat.

Warm-up sequence

When you do yoga, it is important to stretch your body to get it ready. This is called warming up. Here are some poses to warm up your muscles and focus your mind.

Keep your shoulders loose as you move them up and down.

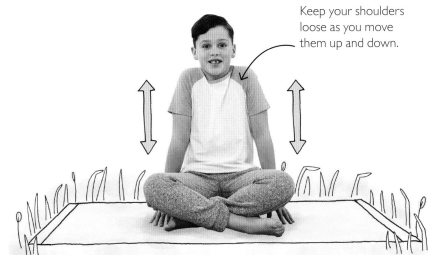

1 Shoulder shrugs

Start with this exercise to loosen up your shoulders. Sit on the floor with your legs crossed and bring your shoulders up to your ears. Then, with a big sigh, let them drop down. Do this three times.

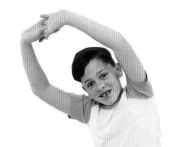

2 Seated side stretch

Next take a big breath in and stretch your arms high above your head. As you breathe out, bend your body and move your arms over to one side. Breathe in and come back to center. Bend to the other side when you breathe out again. Repeat this twice on each side.

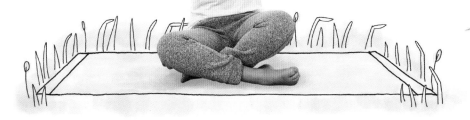

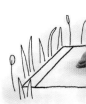

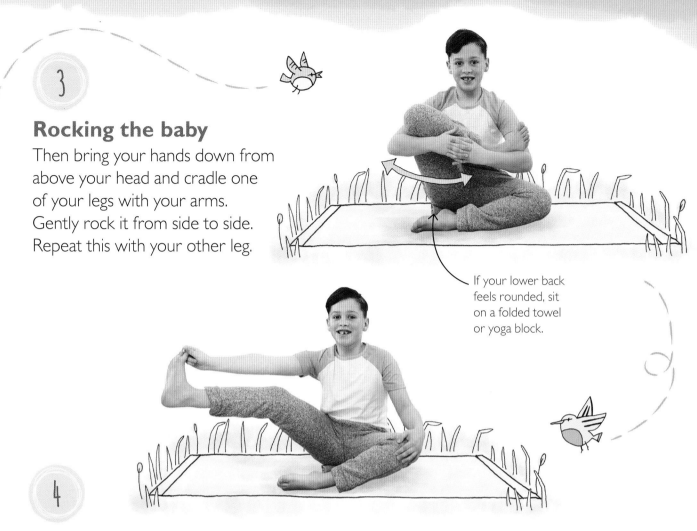

3

Rocking the baby

Then bring your hands down from above your head and cradle one of your legs with your arms. Gently rock it from side to side. Repeat this with your other leg.

If your lower back feels rounded, sit on a folded towel or yoga block.

4

Leg stretch

Once you've rocked your leg, grip the toes of one of your feet and lift your leg out to the side. It doesn't matter if you can't straighten it completely. Bring your leg back in and then do the same on the other side.

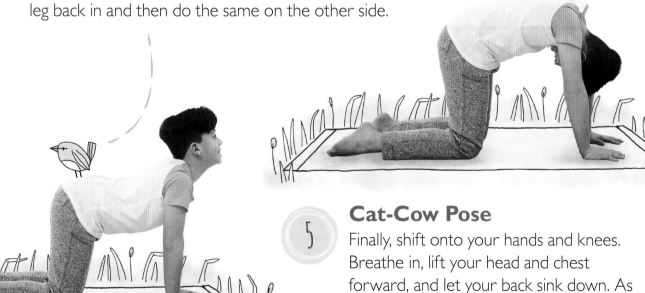

5

Cat-Cow Pose

Finally, shift onto your hands and knees. Breathe in, lift your head and chest forward, and let your back sink down. As you breathe out, round your back and look toward your stomach. Do this three times.

Downward dog

Dogs love giving their bodies a good stretch, and pushing their bodies up into a triangle shape. Can you stretch like a playful pup?

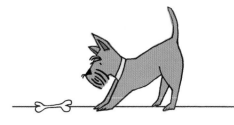

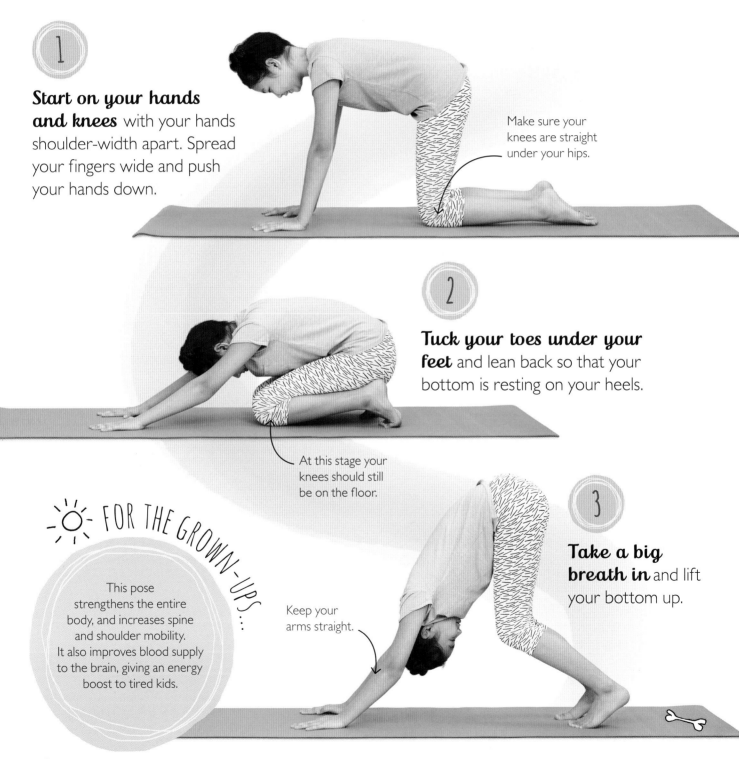

1

Start on your hands and knees with your hands shoulder-width apart. Spread your fingers wide and push your hands down.

Make sure your knees are straight under your hips.

2

Tuck your toes under your feet and lean back so that your bottom is resting on your heels.

At this stage your knees should still be on the floor.

3

Take a big breath in and lift your bottom up.

Keep your arms straight.

☀ FOR THE GROWN-UPS...

This pose strengthens the entire body, and increases spine and shoulder mobility. It also improves blood supply to the brain, giving an energy boost to tired kids.

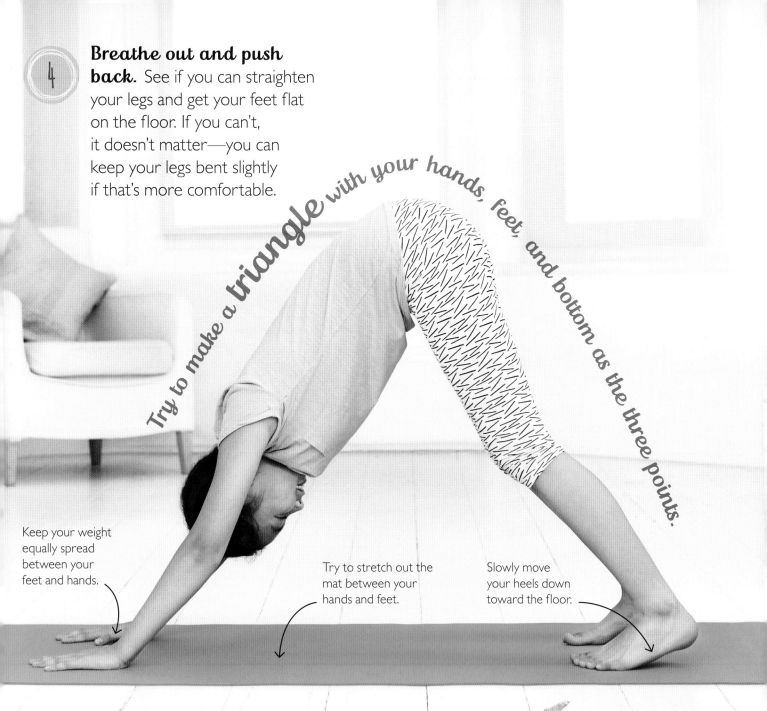

4 **Breathe out and push back.** See if you can straighten your legs and get your feet flat on the floor. If you can't, it doesn't matter—you can keep your legs bent slightly if that's more comfortable.

Try to make a triangle with your hands, feet, and bottom as the three points.

Keep your weight equally spread between your feet and hands.

Try to stretch out the mat between your hands and feet.

Slowly move your heels down toward the floor.

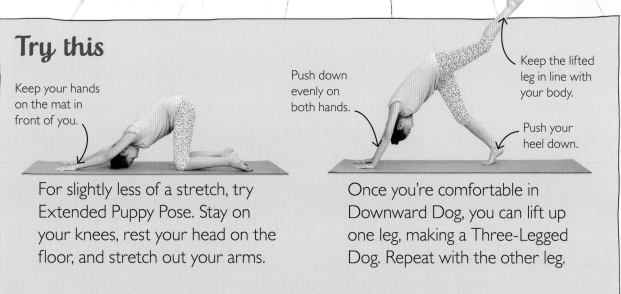

Try this

Keep your hands on the mat in front of you.

For slightly less of a stretch, try Extended Puppy Pose. Stay on your knees, rest your head on the floor, and stretch out your arms.

Push down evenly on both hands.

Keep the lifted leg in line with your body.

Push your heel down.

Once you're comfortable in Downward Dog, you can lift up one leg, making a Three-Legged Dog. Repeat with the other leg.

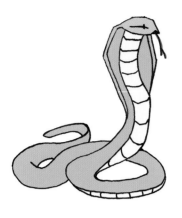

Hissing cobra

When a cobra is giving a warning, it lifts its head and stretches its body up. Can you lift your head high and hiss like a snake?

1 **Start by lying on your front** with your arms crossed under your forehead like a pillow.

Rest your head on your hands.

2 **Move your hands** so your elbows are positioned under your shoulders, then slightly lift up your head. Take a big breath in and hiss as you breathe out.

Be careful not to tense your neck.

Keep your forearms flat on the mat.

This pose increases flexibility of the spine and opens up the chest to improve breathing. Once in the pose, encourage your child to keep their shoulders away from their ears. Slightly bending their arms will help with this.

♫ FOR THE GROWN-UPS...

Try to get the tops of your feet flat on the floor.

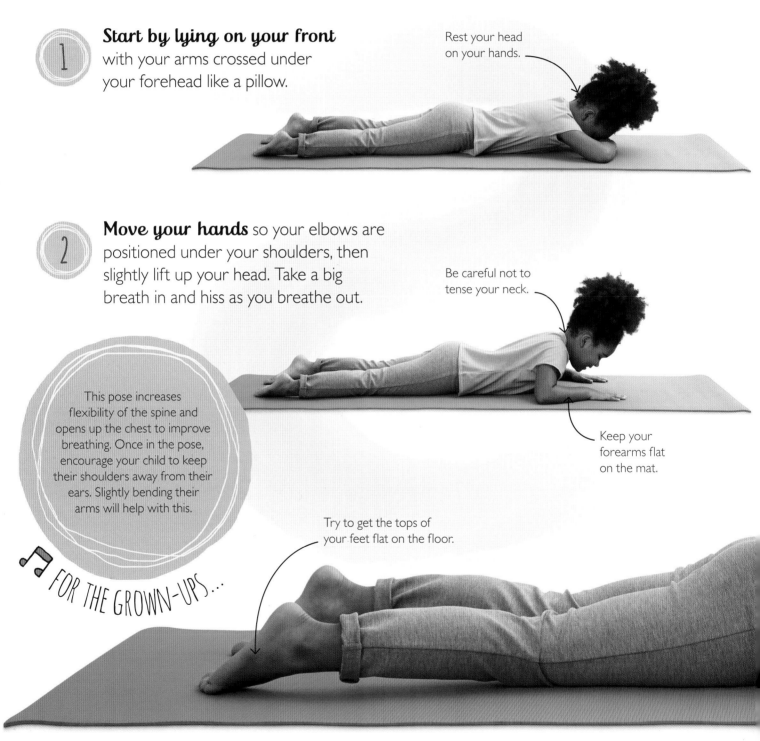

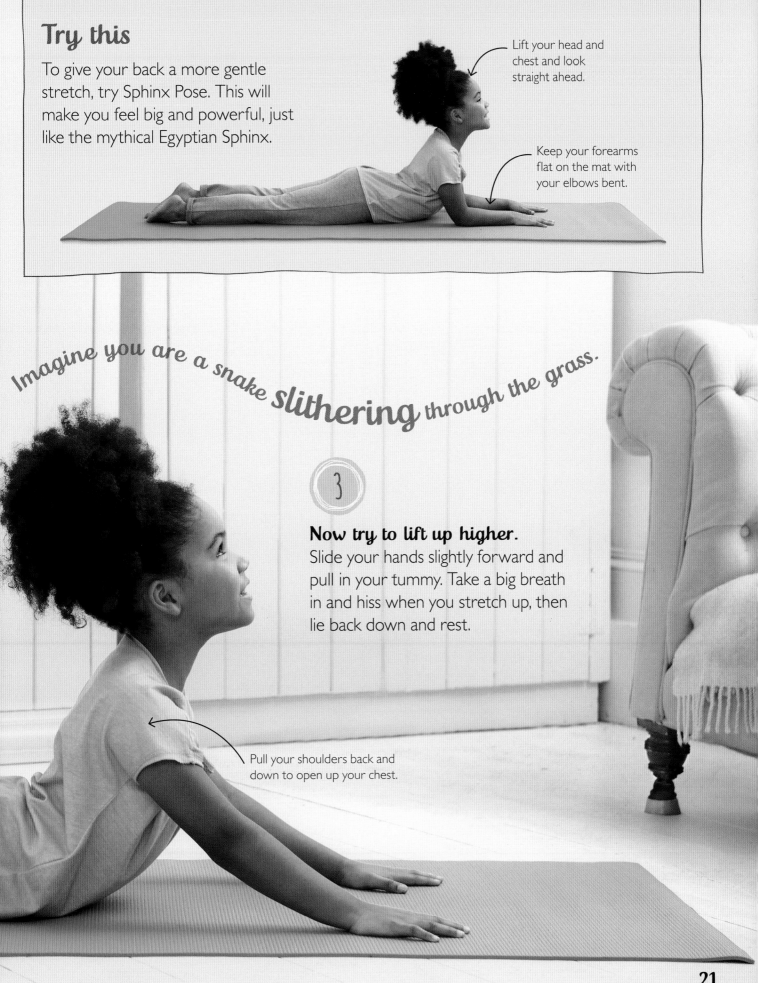

Try this

To give your back a more gentle stretch, try Sphinx Pose. This will make you feel big and powerful, just like the mythical Egyptian Sphinx.

Lift your head and chest and look straight ahead.

Keep your forearms flat on the mat with your elbows bent.

Imagine you are a snake **slithering** through the grass.

③

Now try to lift up higher.
Slide your hands slightly forward and pull in your tummy. Take a big breath in and hiss when you stretch up, then lie back down and rest.

Pull your shoulders back and down to open up your chest.

21

Bendy bow

In this pose, you bend your back to make your body look like the shape of a bow. Imagine your arms and lower legs are the string, ready to shoot an arrow high into the sky.

1 **Lie on your stomach** on your mat. Rest your forehead on the backs of your hands.

Have your legs and feet apart.

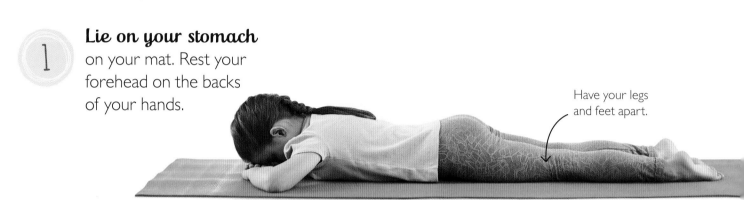

2 **Bend one leg** back and hold your ankle with the hand on the same side as the bent leg.

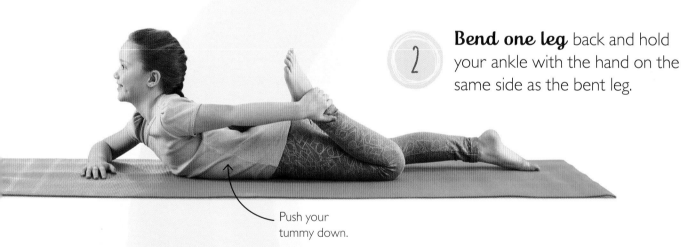

Push your tummy down.

3 **Bend the other leg** and hold the ankle with your other hand.

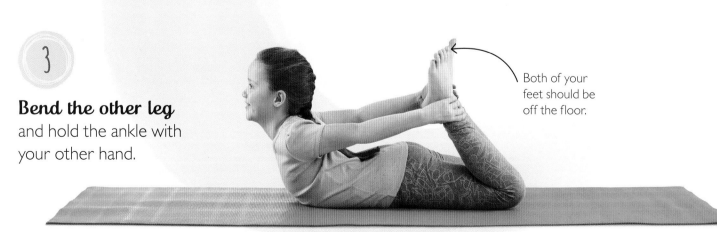

Both of your feet should be off the floor.

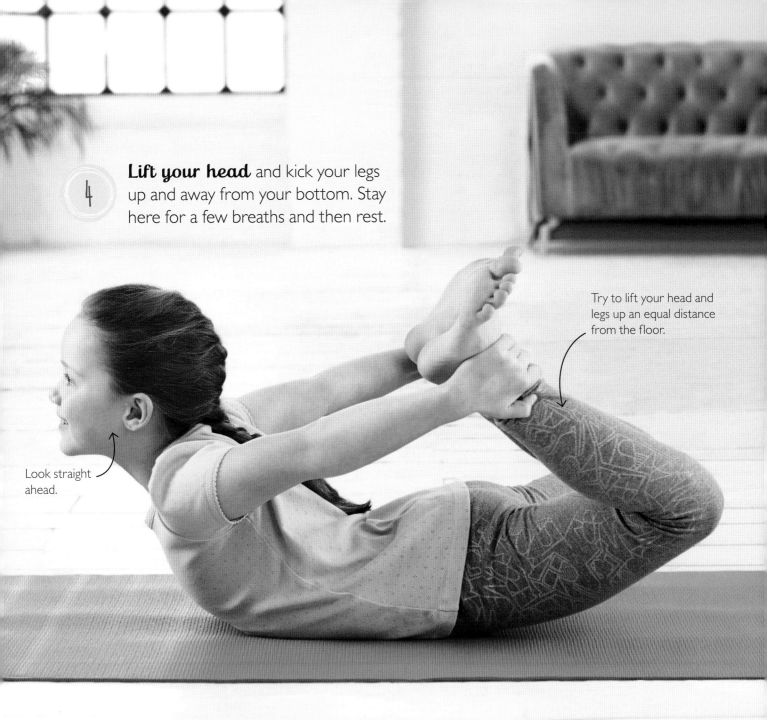

4 **Lift your head** and kick your legs up and away from your bottom. Stay here for a few breaths and then rest.

Try to lift your head and legs up an equal distance from the floor.

Look straight ahead.

Try this

If it's difficult to lift your legs, just lift your head and body.

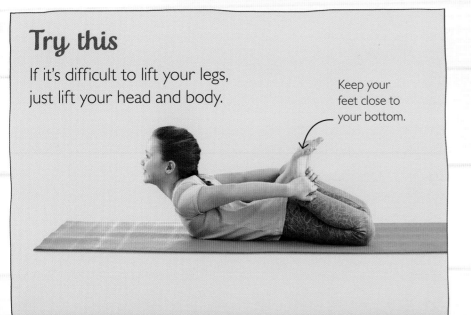

Keep your feet close to your bottom.

● FOR THE GROWN-UPS…

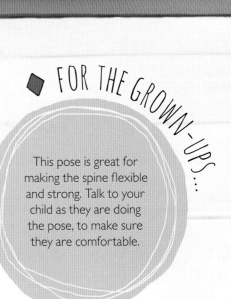

This pose is great for making the spine flexible and strong. Talk to your child as they are doing the pose, to make sure they are comfortable.

Lion's breath

When a tired lion yawns, it opens its mouth wide and stretches out its tongue. Pretend to be a lion and wake up your face with this playful pose.

FOR THE GROWN-UPS...

This pose is great for relieving tension in the face and chest. It also helps to strengthen the voice and encourages kids to be more confident when speaking and singing.

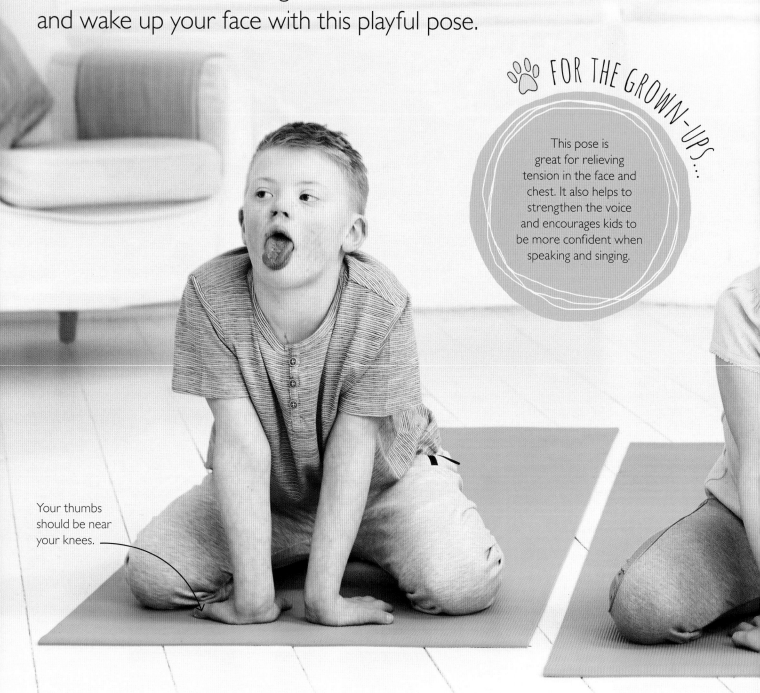

Your thumbs should be near your knees.

 Start by kneeling with your bottom on your heels, your big toes together, and your knees apart. Lean forward and put your strong lion paws on the floor. Turn your hands backward so that your fingers are pointing toward you.

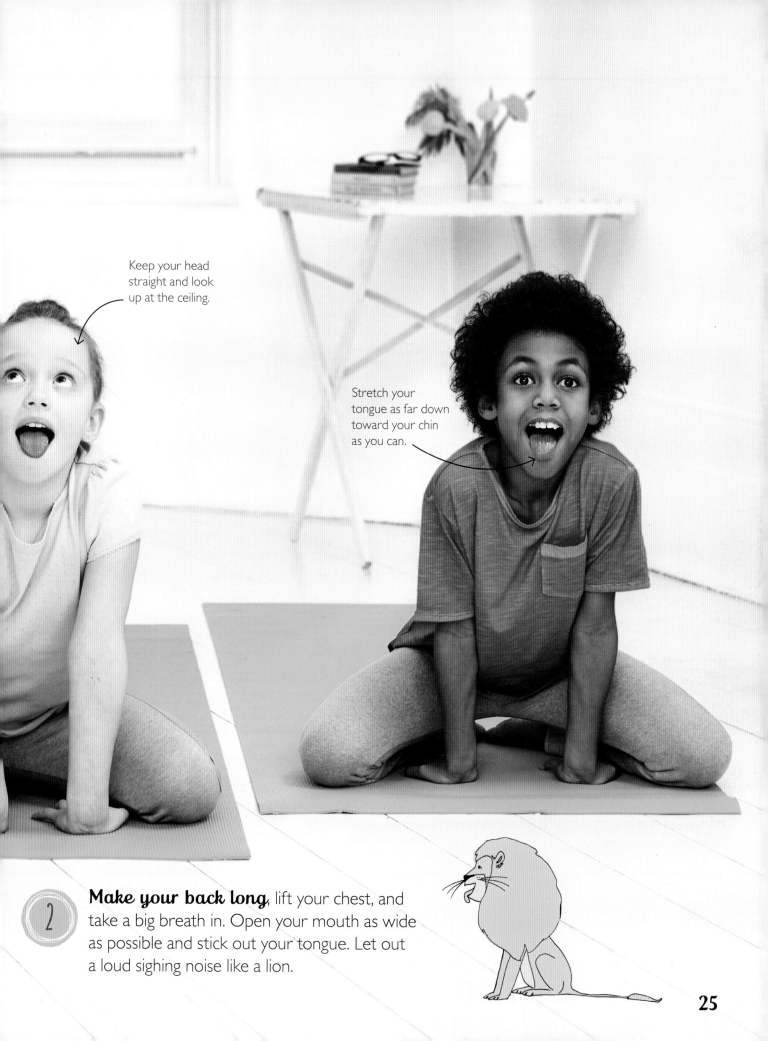

Keep your head straight and look up at the ceiling.

Stretch your tongue as far down toward your chin as you can.

2 **Make your back long**, lift your chest, and take a big breath in. Open your mouth as wide as possible and stick out your tongue. Let out a loud sighing noise like a lion.

25

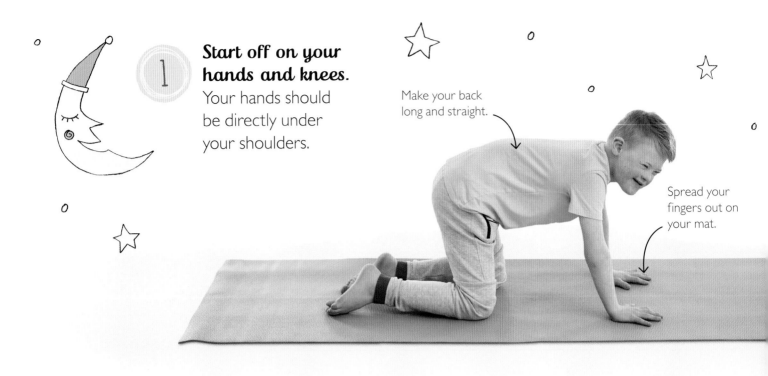

1 **Start off on your hands and knees.** Your hands should be directly under your shoulders.

Make your back long and straight.

Spread your fingers out on your mat.

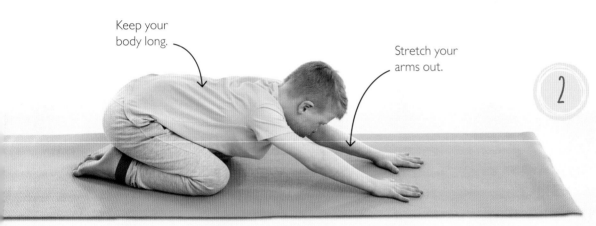

Keep your body long.

Stretch your arms out.

2 **Bring your bottom** down so that it rests on your heels. Slide your hands out in front of you.

Resting child

Have you ever noticed how peaceful babies look when they sleep? Child's Pose helps you to feel as relaxed as a sleeping baby. It's a great way to rest your body and calm down your breathing.

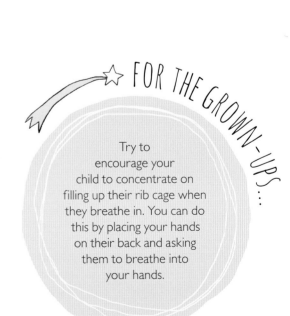

FOR THE GROWN-UPS...

Try to encourage your child to concentrate on filling up their rib cage when they breathe in. You can do this by placing your hands on their back and asking them to breathe into your hands.

Rest your forehead on the mat. Bring your arms down next to your sides, and close your eyes. When you're ready, slowly come out of the pose.

3

Focus on your **breathing**. How does it **feel** and **sound?**

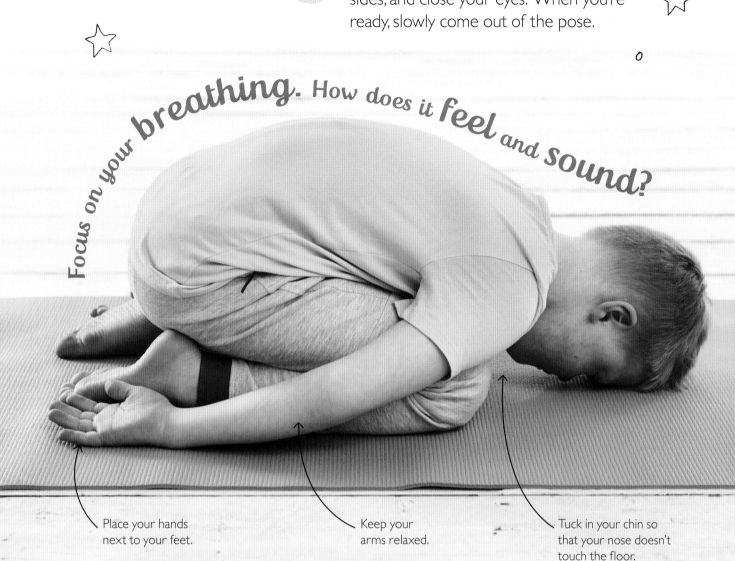

Place your hands next to your feet.

Keep your arms relaxed.

Tuck in your chin so that your nose doesn't touch the floor.

Try this

If you want to give your arms and back a stretch, put your hands out in front of you.

Push your hands into the mat to move your bottom toward your heels.

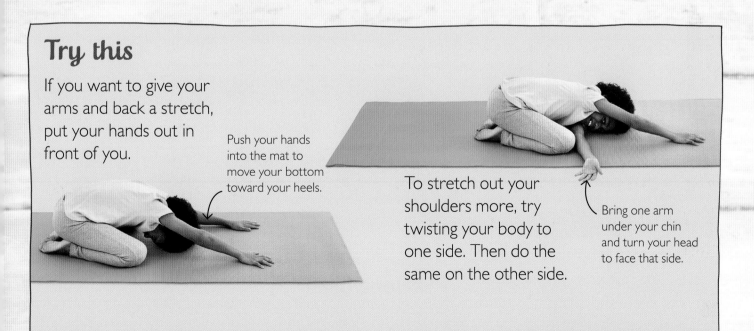

To stretch out your shoulders more, try twisting your body to one side. Then do the same on the other side.

Bring one arm under your chin and turn your head to face that side.

Sailing boat

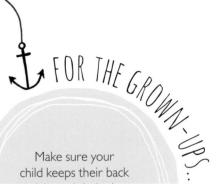

This pose will help make all the muscles in your body stronger. It's particularly good for your tummy muscles and your balance.

FOR THE GROWN-UPS...

Make sure your child keeps their back straight and their chest lifted, to stop them from rolling backward.

Sit down and hug your knees close to you. Keep your back straight.

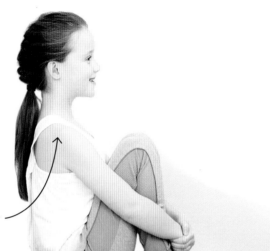

Keep your shoulders as far from your ears as you can.

Keep the back of your neck long.

Lift your chest.

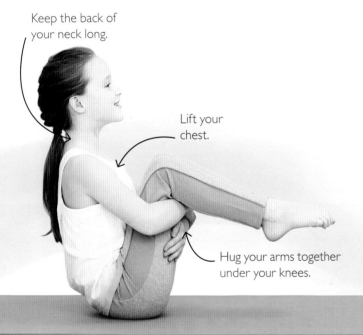

Hug your arms together under your knees.

Lean back slightly and lift your heels off the floor, then lift your toes, too. Make sure you keep your back straight and the top of your head lifted up.

This pose is meant to make you look like a small **boat**. Your back is

3 **Lift up your feet** and stretch out your arms so that they are next to your legs. Looking at your feet can help you balance. See how long you can stay in this position without falling over.

Try this

Your tummy muscles should feel tight because they are helping you balance.

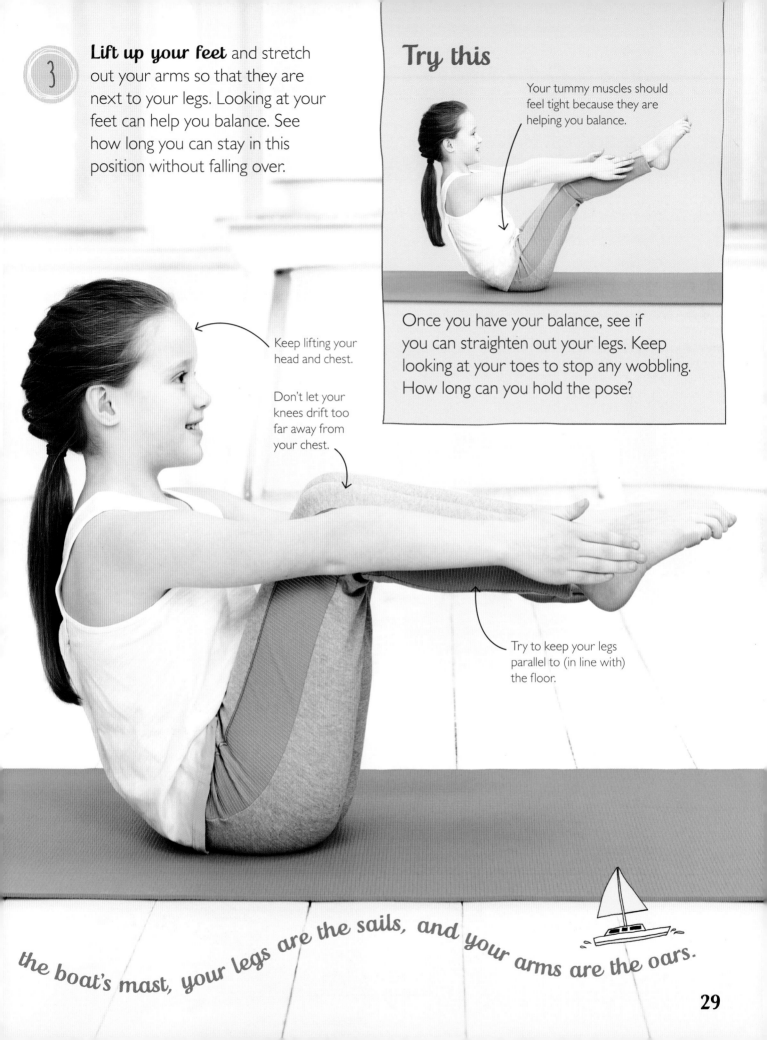

Once you have your balance, see if you can straighten out your legs. Keep looking at your toes to stop any wobbling. How long can you hold the pose?

Keep lifting your head and chest.

Don't let your knees drift too far away from your chest.

Try to keep your legs parallel to (in line with) the floor.

the boat's mast, your legs are the sails, and your arms are the oars.

Energetic sequence

It is normal to feel tired and worn out from time to time. This sequence is great for helping you feel full of energy.

1

Downward Dog

Start on your hands and knees and lift your bottom up into the air into Downward Dog. Keep your arms strong, your fingers spread out, and push your body toward your legs. Stay here for five breaths.

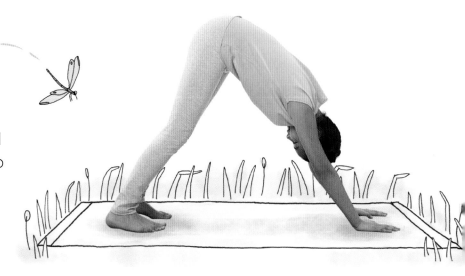

2

Table

Next lower your knees to the mat so that you're on your hands and knees again. Then lie down on your front.

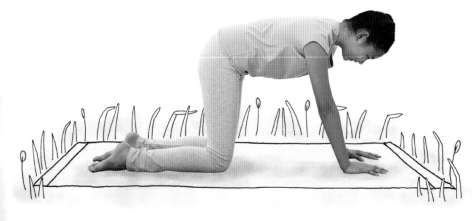

3

Cobra

Now put your hands on the floor in front of your shoulders and slowly peel yourself up into Cobra Pose. Do this twice, resting for a few moments in between and when you've finished.

Slowly lift yourself up off your yoga mat.

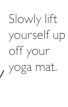

Bow

Bend both your legs and hold your ankles. Keep your head and chest lifted and kick your feet back and up toward the ceiling. Stay here for three to five breaths and then kneel.

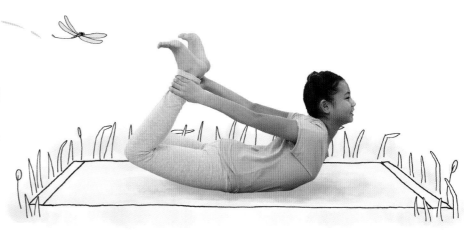

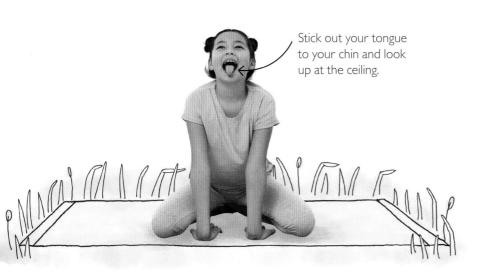

Stick out your tongue to your chin and look up at the ceiling.

Lion

Spread your knees wide but keep your big toes touching. Put your hands on the floor, fingers pointing back to your toes. As you breathe out, make a noisy lion sigh. Repeat this three times.

Namaste

Finally, sit with your legs crossed and eyes closed. Think about how you are breathing, then bring your hands together into Namaste position.

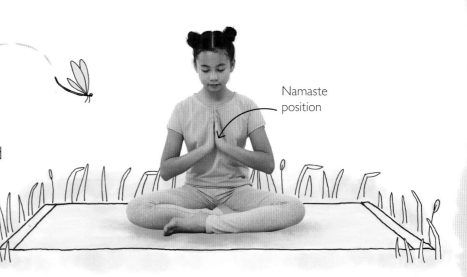

Namaste position

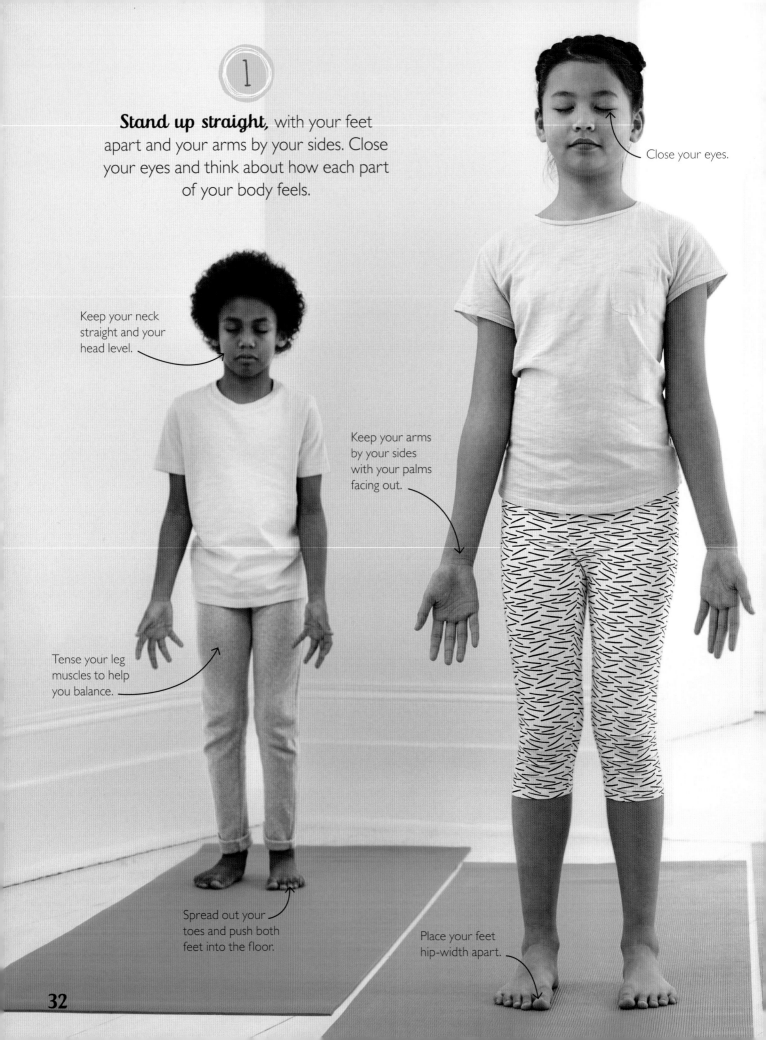

Stand up straight, with your feet apart and your arms by your sides. Close your eyes and think about how each part of your body feels.

Close your eyes.

Keep your neck straight and your head level.

Keep your arms by your sides with your palms facing out.

Tense your leg muscles to help you balance.

Spread out your toes and push both feet into the floor.

Place your feet hip-width apart.

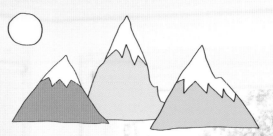

Mighty mountain

This is one of the most important poses in yoga. It relaxes the mind and teaches you to be still and strong, just like a mighty mountain.

Pull your tummy in and stand up straight.

This pose is great for making kids aware of their posture. Make sure that your child stands tall and strong with their shoulders down while they focus on their breathing.

FOR THE GROWN-UPS...

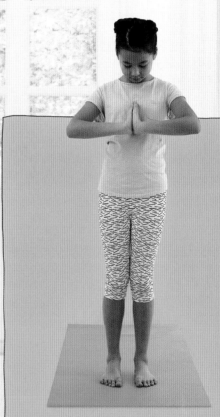

Try this

When you're ready to come out of Mountain Pose, breathe in and bring your arms above your head with your hands touching. When you breathe out, bring your hands in front of your chest into Namaste.

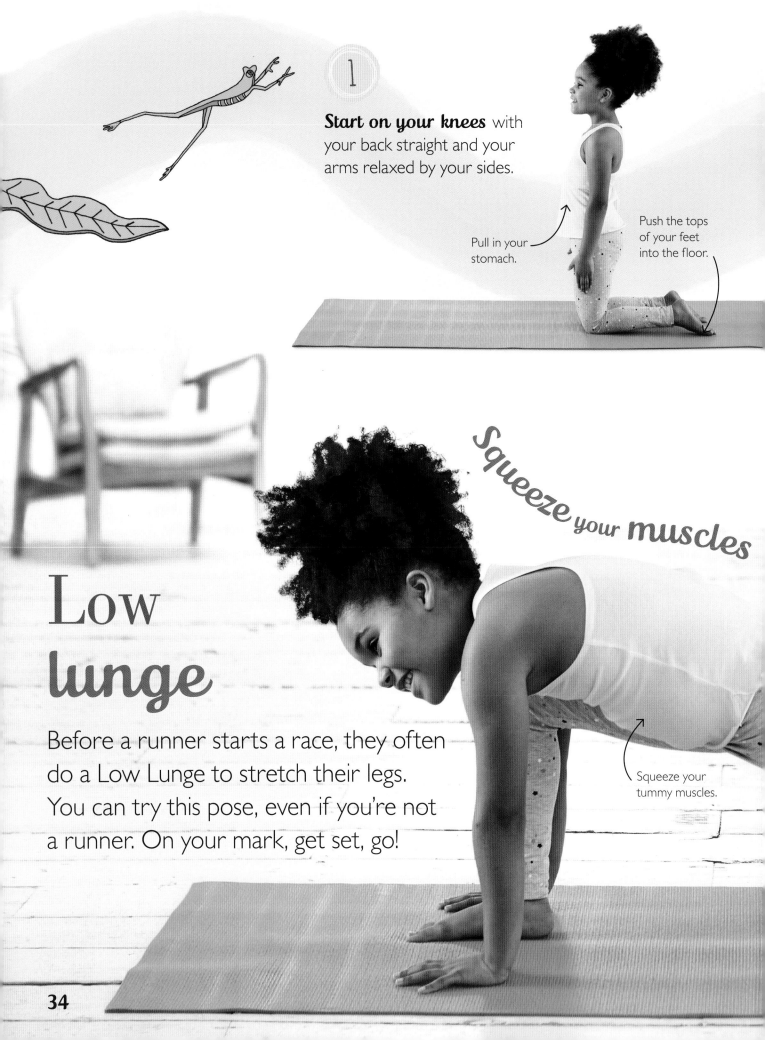

Start on your knees with your back straight and your arms relaxed by your sides.

Pull in your stomach.

Push the tops of your feet into the floor.

Squeeze your muscles

Squeeze your tummy muscles.

Low lunge

Before a runner starts a race, they often do a Low Lunge to stretch their legs. You can try this pose, even if you're not a runner. On your mark, get set, go!

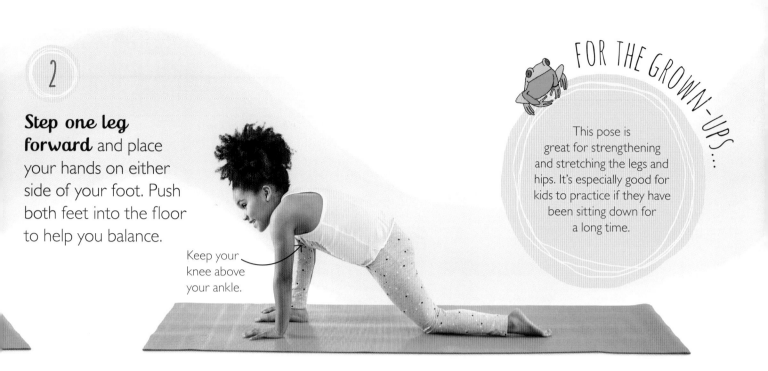

2

Step one leg forward and place your hands on either side of your foot. Push both feet into the floor to help you balance.

Keep your knee above your ankle.

FOR THE GROWN-UPS...

This pose is great for strengthening and stretching the legs and hips. It's especially good for kids to practice if they have been sitting down for a long time.

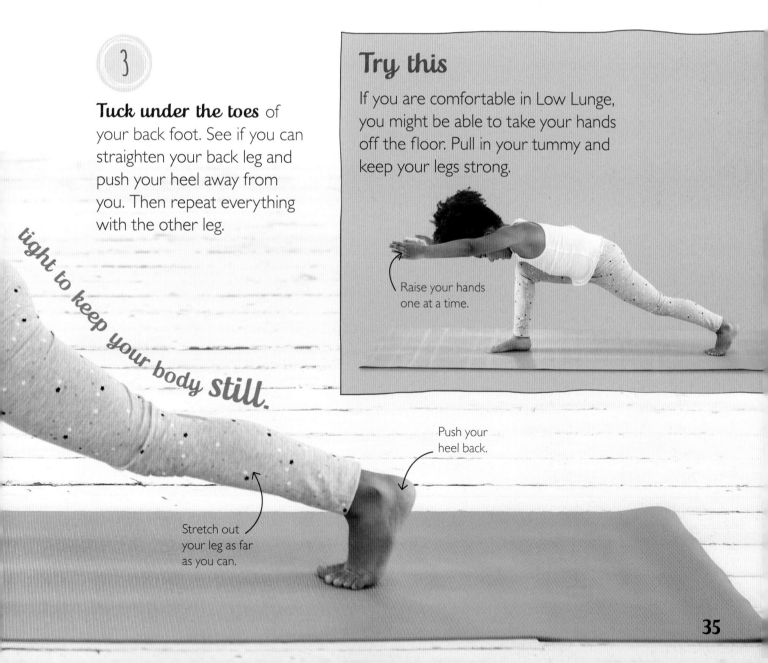

3

Tuck under the toes of your back foot. See if you can straighten your back leg and push your heel away from you. Then repeat everything with the other leg.

tight to keep your body still.

Try this

If you are comfortable in Low Lunge, you might be able to take your hands off the floor. Pull in your tummy and keep your legs strong.

Raise your hands one at a time.

Push your heel back.

Stretch out your leg as far as you can.

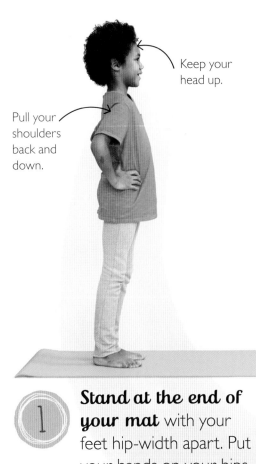

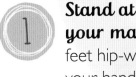
Pull your shoulders back and down.

Keep your head up.

Mighty warrior

Warrior 1 Pose warms you up, gives you energy, and makes you strong. Stand up tall, put your hands on your hips, and prepare for victory!

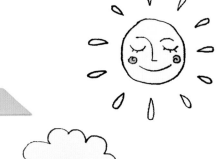

1 Stand at the end of your mat with your feet hip-width apart. Put your hands on your hips.

Keep your left leg and foot facing forward.

2 Turn out the toes of your right foot, then take a big step forward with your left foot.

Don't stick out your bottom.

Push your heel into the floor.

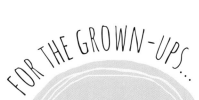
FOR THE GROWN-UPS...

This energizing pose strengthens the whole body, from the ankles up to the back and arms. It helps to improve focus, balance, and stability.

3 Breathe out and bend your front knee so it is right over the top of your ankle. Press down into your back foot.

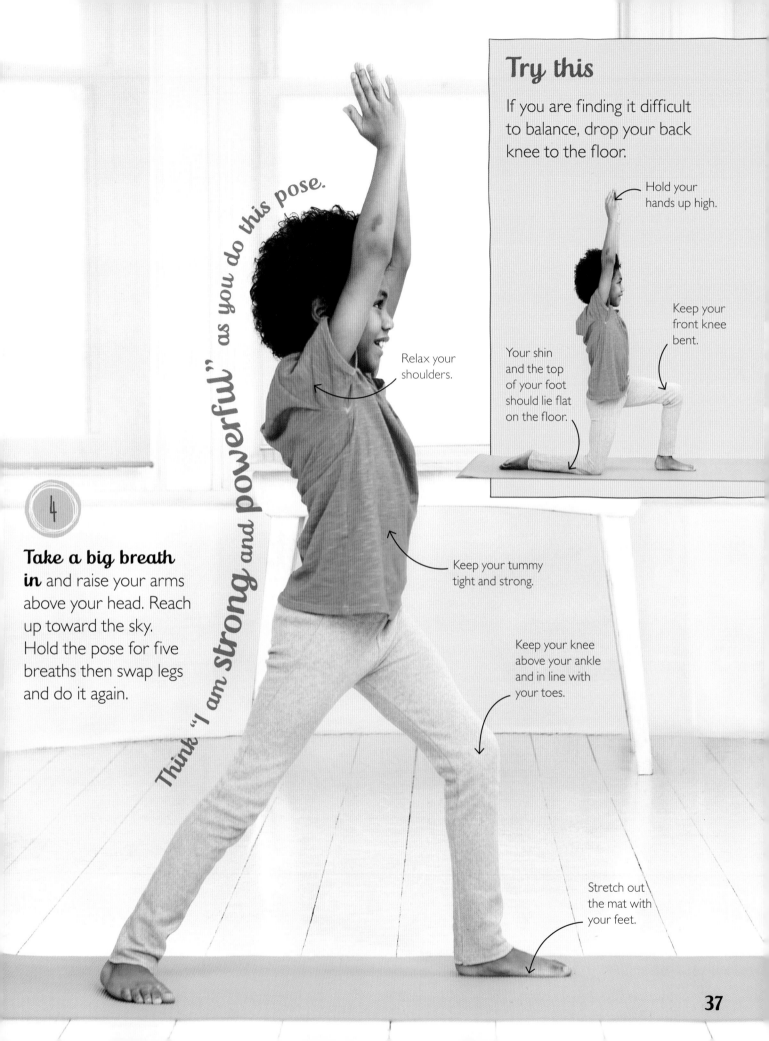

Think "I am **strong** and **powerful**" as you do this pose.

Try this

If you are finding it difficult to balance, drop your back knee to the floor.

Hold your hands up high.

Keep your front knee bent.

Your shin and the top of your foot should lie flat on the floor.

4

Take a big breath in and raise your arms above your head. Reach up toward the sky. Hold the pose for five breaths then swap legs and do it again.

Relax your shoulders.

Keep your tummy tight and strong.

Keep your knee above your ankle and in line with your toes.

Stretch out the mat with your feet.

Invisible chair

Amaze your friends by sitting on an invisible chair. This pose will keep your legs strong.

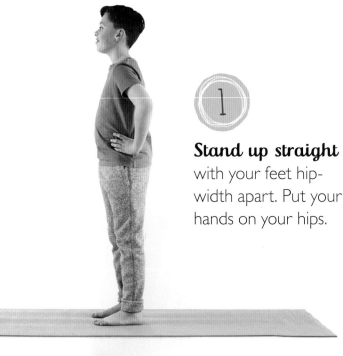

1

Stand up straight with your feet hip-width apart. Put your hands on your hips.

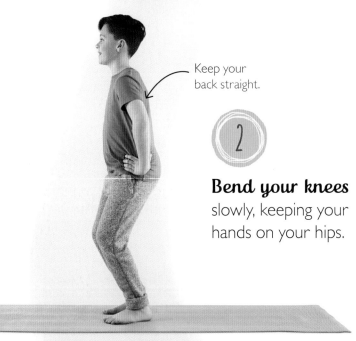

Keep your back straight.

2

Bend your knees slowly, keeping your hands on your hips.

Don't arch your back.

Look down toward your feet.

3

Push your hips back and tilt your body forward.

FOR THE GROWN-UPS...

This pose tones the muscles in the thighs and calves, and strengthens the hips. It's also a great way to help correct bad posture and stop your child from slouching.

Try this

To strengthen your legs, try doing Chair Pose against a wall. Push your back into the wall and your feet into the floor.

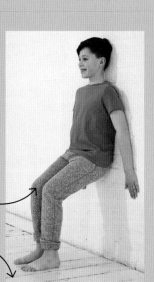

Stand with your feet and knees hip-width apart.

Don't use a mat for this because it could slip out from underneath you.

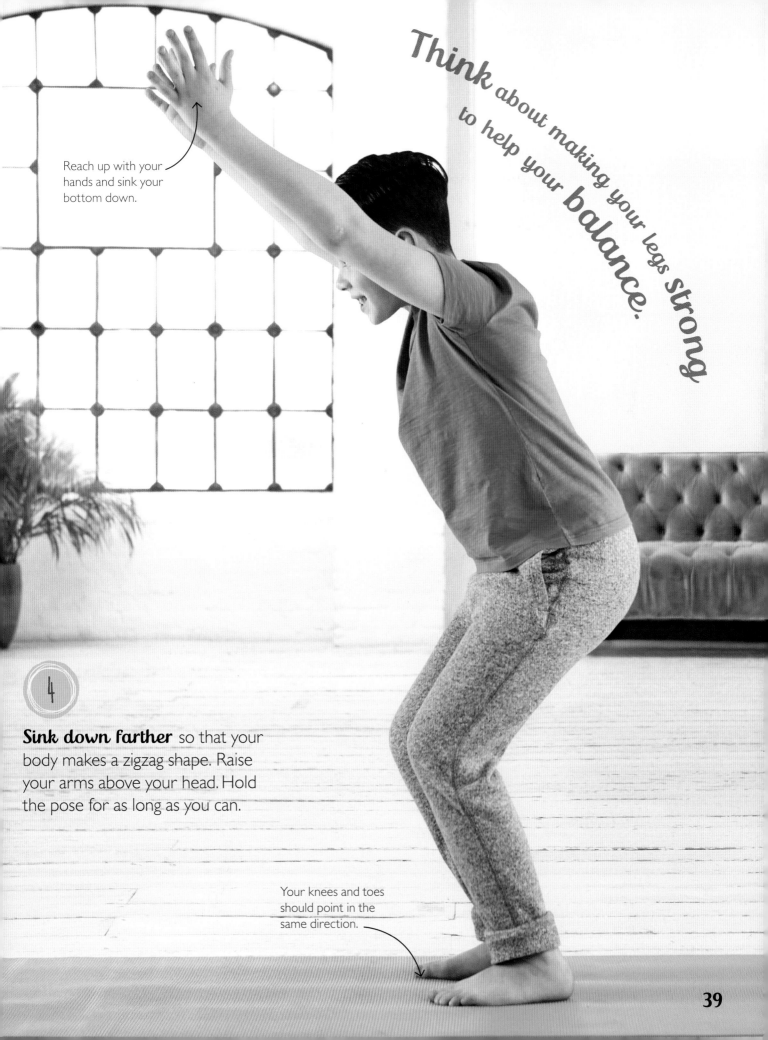

Reach up with your hands and sink your bottom down.

4

Sink down farther so that your body makes a zigzag shape. Raise your arms above your head. Hold the pose for as long as you can.

Your knees and toes should point in the same direction.

39

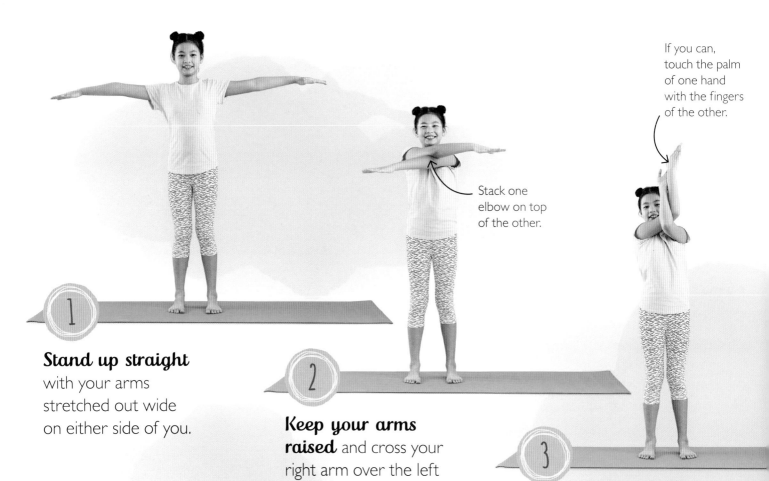

Stand up straight with your arms stretched out wide on either side of you.

Keep your arms raised and cross your right arm over the left in front of your chest.

Stack one elbow on top of the other.

If you can, touch the palm of one hand with the fingers of the other.

Bend your arms up toward your face and wrap them around each other. One hand should be higher than the other.

Twisted eagle

Wrap your arms and legs around each other in this twisty balancing pose. You'll feel as powerful as an eagle after this whole body stretch.

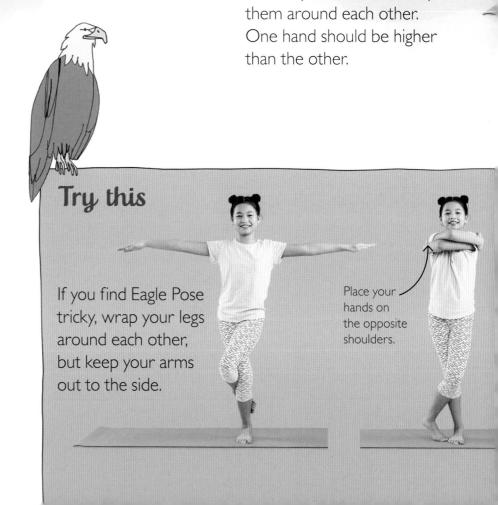

Try this

If you find Eagle Pose tricky, wrap your legs around each other, but keep your arms out to the side.

Place your hands on the opposite shoulders.

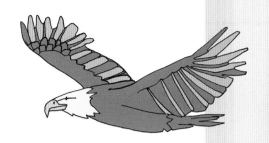

Reach up with
your fingers.

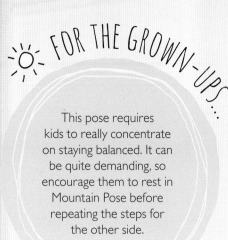
FOR THE GROWN-UPS...

This pose requires
kids to really concentrate
on staying balanced. It can
be quite demanding, so
encourage them to rest in
Mountain Pose before
repeating the steps for
the other side.

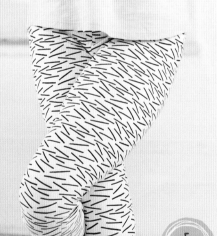

Keep your
elbows lifted.

Pull in your stomach and
squeeze your legs together
to help you balance.

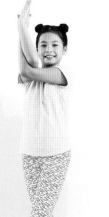

4

**Keeping your arms
wrapped** around each
other, lift your left leg and
cross it over your right leg.

If you're finding it
hard to balance,
cross one leg over
the other and rest
your foot on the
floor. Cross your
arms in front of you.

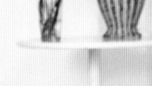

5

Lift up your left foot and
tuck it behind your right calf.
Stay in this position for a few
breaths. Then repeat steps
one to five for the other side.

41

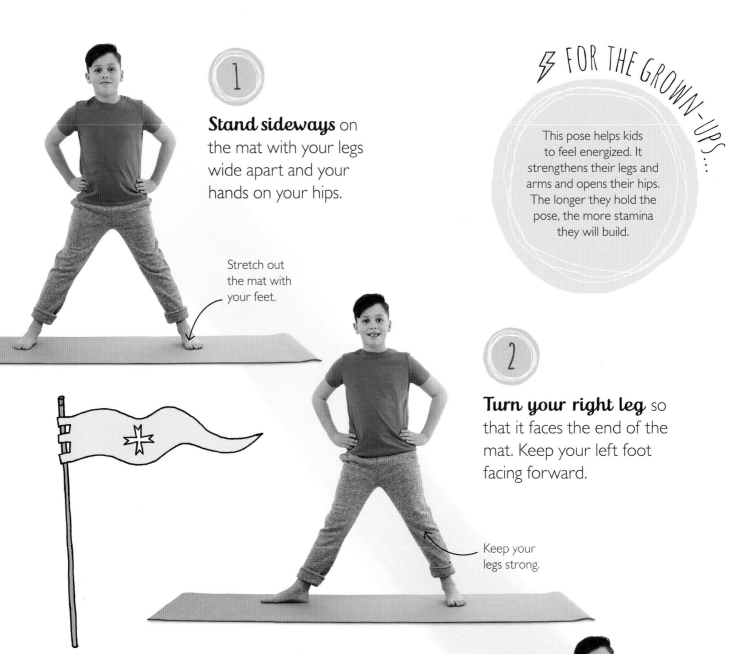

Stand sideways on the mat with your legs wide apart and your hands on your hips.

Stretch out the mat with your feet.

2

Turn your right leg so that it faces the end of the mat. Keep your left foot facing forward.

Keep your legs strong.

Stretching warrior

The yoga warrior is strong and powerful. Try Warrior II Pose for yourself. Do you feel like a mighty warrior?

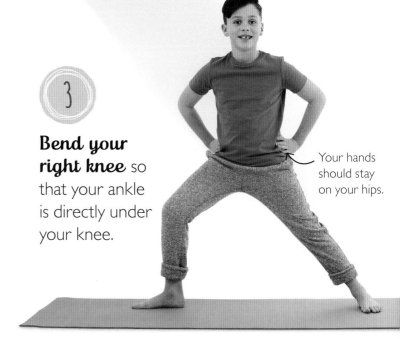

3

Bend your right knee so that your ankle is directly under your knee.

Your hands should stay on your hips.

This pose is also called "Surfer" because it looks like you're on a surfboard!

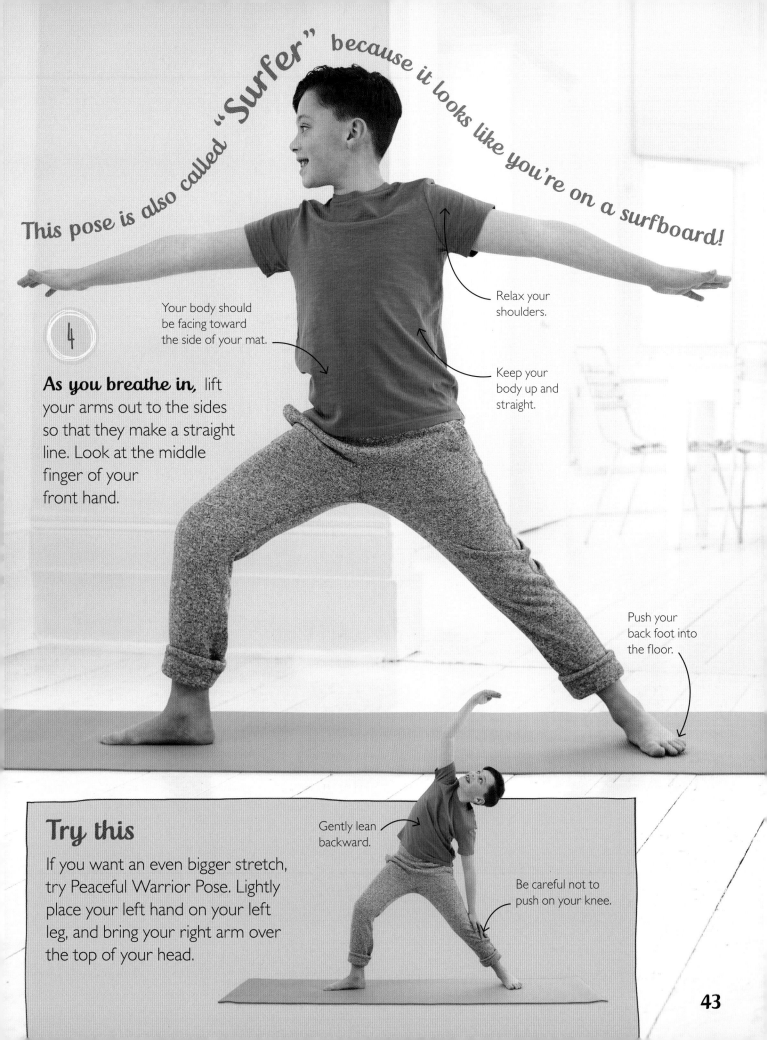

Relax your shoulders.

Your body should be facing toward the side of your mat.

Keep your body up and straight.

4

As you breathe in, lift your arms out to the sides so that they make a straight line. Look at the middle finger of your front hand.

Push your back foot into the floor.

Try this

If you want an even bigger stretch, try Peaceful Warrior Pose. Lightly place your left hand on your left leg, and bring your right arm over the top of your head.

Gently lean backward.

Be careful not to push on your knee.

43

Confidence sequence

Try this sequence to make you feel strong, powerful, and confident.

1

Mountain

Start by facing sideways on your mat with your legs wide apart. Place your hands on your hips.

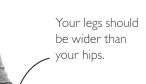

Your legs should be wider than your hips.

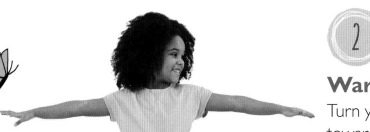

2

Warrior II

Turn your left foot out to point toward the front of the mat and bend your left knee. Bring your arms up and out to the sides. Hold for a few breaths, then repeat with the other leg.

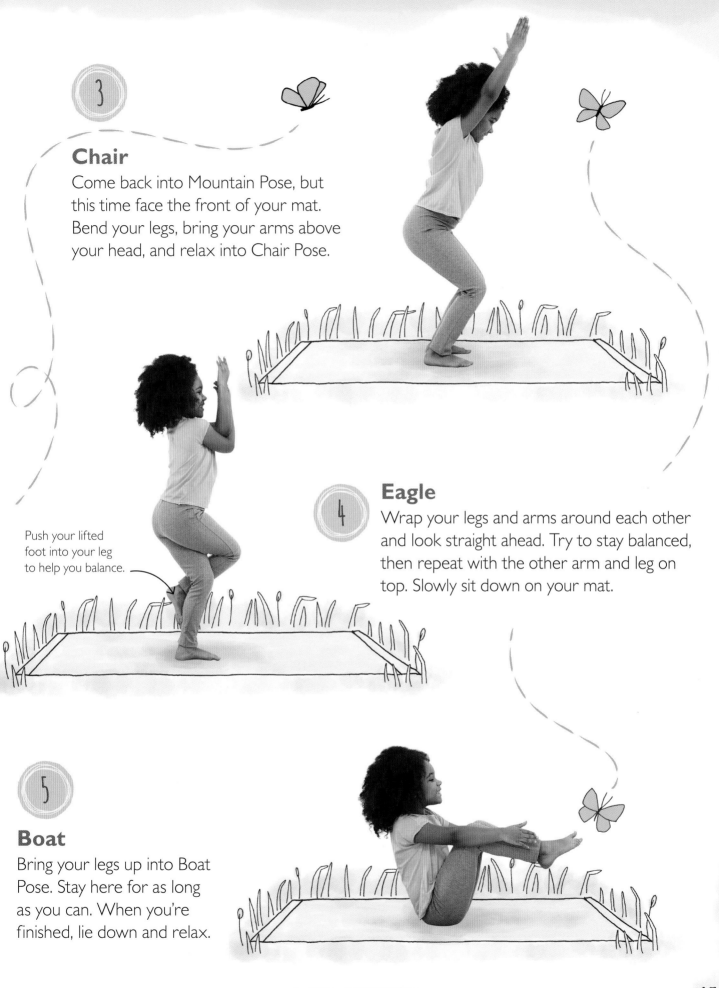

Chair

3

Come back into Mountain Pose, but this time face the front of your mat. Bend your legs, bring your arms above your head, and relax into Chair Pose.

Push your lifted foot into your leg to help you balance.

Eagle

4

Wrap your legs and arms around each other and look straight ahead. Try to stay balanced, then repeat with the other arm and leg on top. Slowly sit down on your mat.

Boat

5

Bring your legs up into Boat Pose. Stay here for as long as you can. When you're finished, lie down and relax.

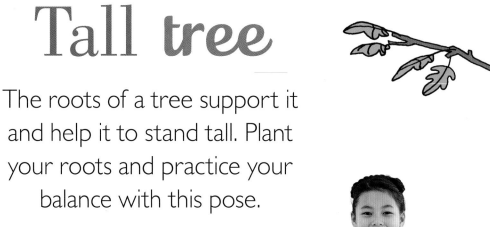

Tall tree

The roots of a tree support it and help it to stand tall. Plant your roots and practice your balance with this pose.

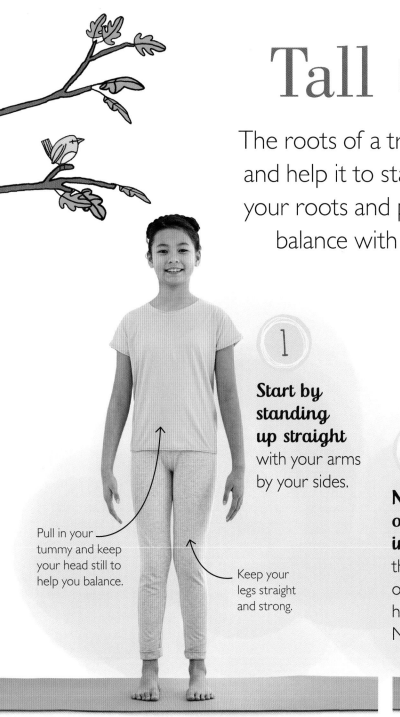

1

Start by standing up straight with your arms by your sides.

Pull in your tummy and keep your head still to help you balance.

Keep your legs straight and strong.

2

Now imagine that one foot is planted into the ground. Put the other foot on top of it and bring your hands together into Namaste position.

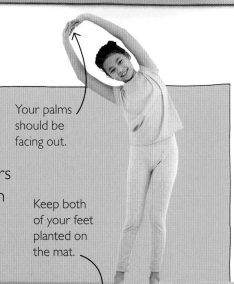

Try this

If you're finding it hard to balance, try Swaying Palm Tree Pose. Link your fingers together, stretch your arms up straight in the air, and bend over to one side. Then bend over to the other side.

Your palms should be facing out.

Keep both of your feet planted on the mat.

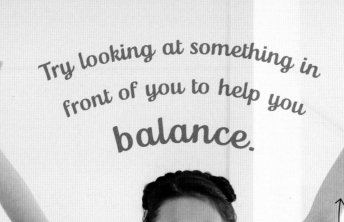

Try looking at something in front of you to help you **balance.**

Stretch your arms up and out above your head, as if they were branches.

3

If your balance is good today, you can try bringing your lifted foot higher on your leg. Push your foot and your leg into each other and count how long you can stay here. When you've finished, try the pose again on the other side.

You can use your hand to help pull up your foot.

 FOR THE GROWN-UPS ...

Balance is affected by how busy our minds are, so it can be different every day and at different times of day. If your child struggles, let them know they are doing well for that particular time or day.

Press your lifted foot into your standing leg. Make sure it is above or below your knee, not on your knee.

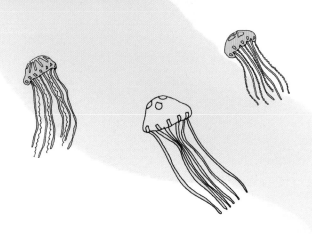

Standing forward bend

What does the world look like when you're upside down? Find out in this pose, where you can dangle your arms like jellyfish tentacles!

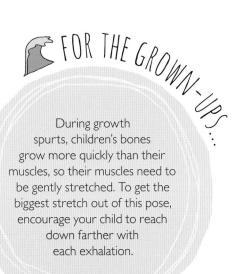

FOR THE GROWN-UPS...

During growth spurts, children's bones grow more quickly than their muscles, so their muscles need to be gently stretched. To get the biggest stretch out of this pose, encourage your child to reach down farther with each exhalation.

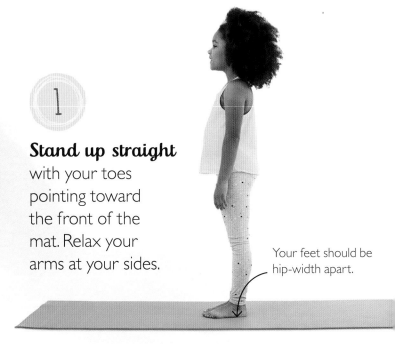

1

Stand up straight with your toes pointing toward the front of the mat. Relax your arms at your sides.

Your feet should be hip-width apart.

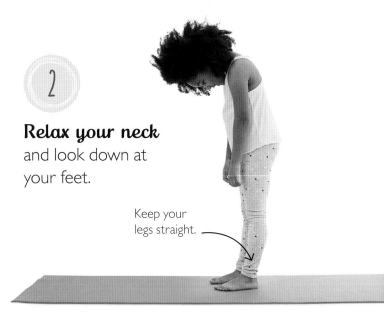

2

Relax your neck and look down at your feet.

Keep your legs straight.

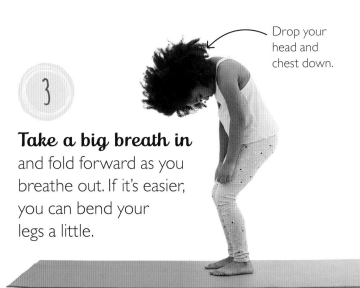

Drop your head and chest down.

3

Take a big breath in and fold forward as you breathe out. If it's easier, you can bend your legs a little.

Try this

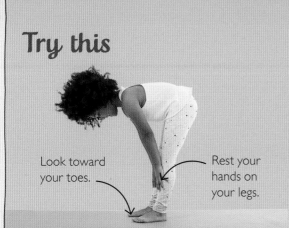

Look toward your toes.

Rest your hands on your legs.

For a different stretch, come up halfway and make your back and neck as straight as you can.

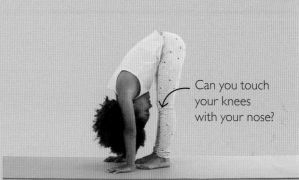

Can you touch your knees with your nose?

If you're comfortable upside down, try straightening your legs for a deeper stretch.

4

Stretch down as far as you can and try to touch the mat with your hands. Stay here for a few breaths, then slowly roll your body back up to standing. Your head should be the last thing to come up.

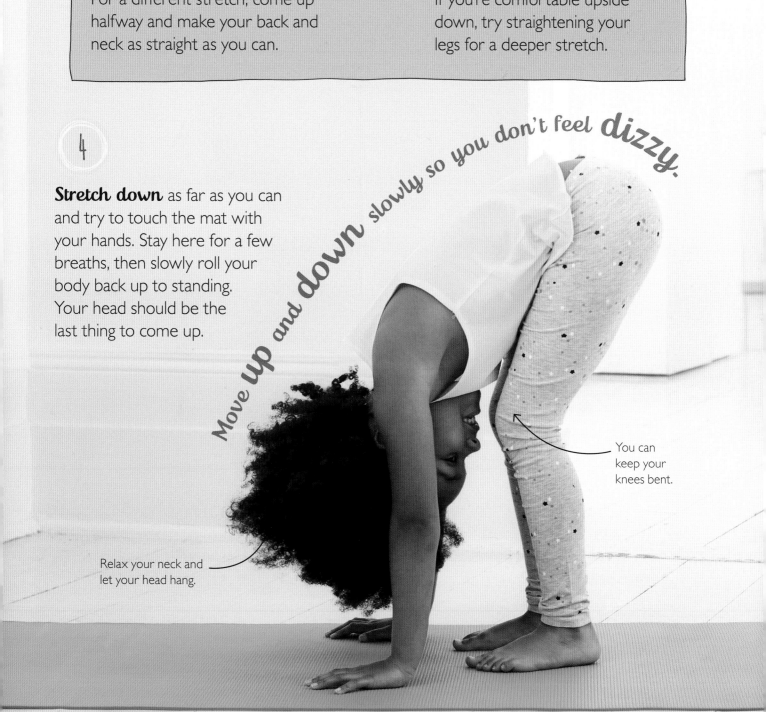

Move **up and down** slowly so you don't feel **dizzy.**

You can keep your knees bent.

Relax your neck and let your head hang.

Happy baby

Babies are very playful. They enjoy holding their feet and rocking on their backs. This pose can be great fun for older kids, too. Why don't you give it a try?

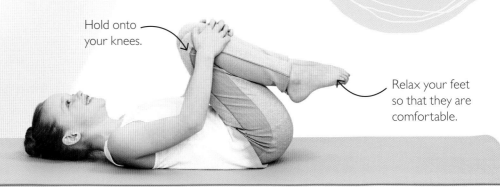

Hold onto your knees.

Relax your feet so that they are comfortable.

1 **Lie on your back on the mat.** Breathe in, then out, and bend your knees into your tummy.

Touch your big toes together.

Relax your neck and keep your head on the floor.

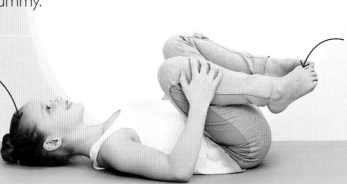

2 **Breathe in** and open your knees so that they are wider than your body. Bring them up toward your armpits.

Try this

If you find Happy Baby easy, try it again with your legs out straight. Hold your shins as you rock from side to side.

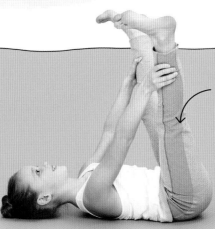

Make your legs as straight as possible.

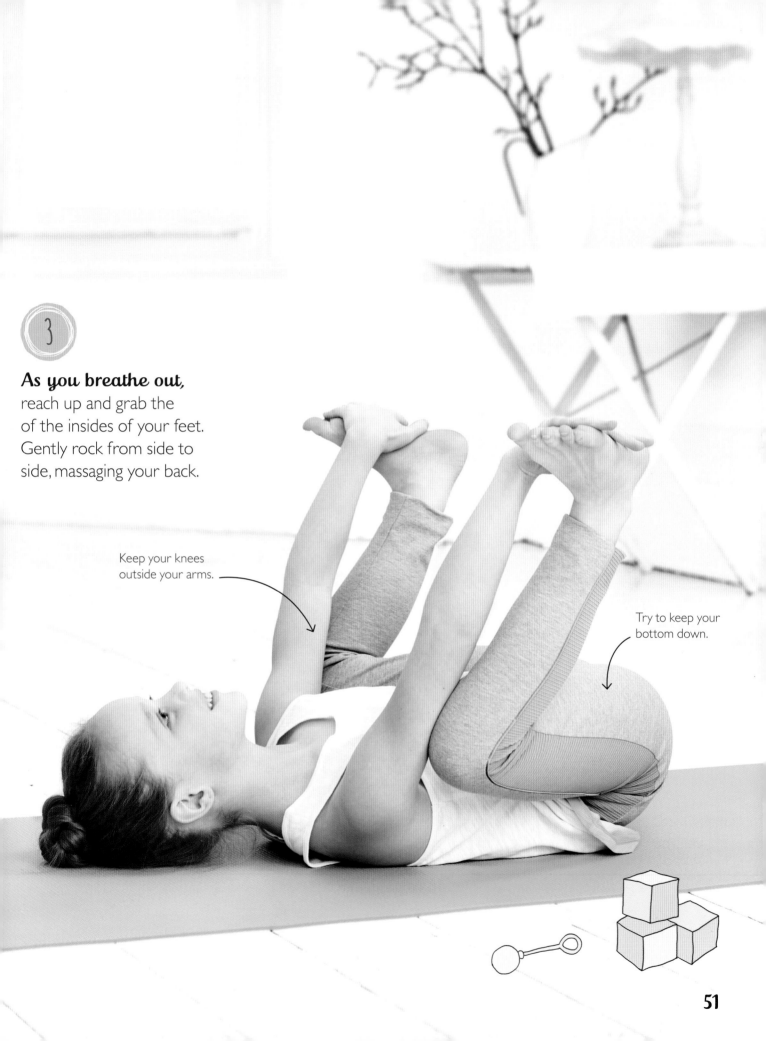

3

As you breathe out,
reach up and grab the
of the insides of your feet.
Gently rock from side to
side, massaging your back.

Keep your knees
outside your arms.

Try to keep your
bottom down.

51

Sit in a comfortable position with your legs crossed. Take a big breath in through your nose and fill your whole body up with air, like a balloon.

Put one finger on your lips and make a humming sound like a bee as you breathe out. This should make your lips tingle.

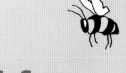

Humming bee breath

This breathing exercise will make you sound like a buzzy bumblebee! Follow these steps whenever your brain feels busy or tired.

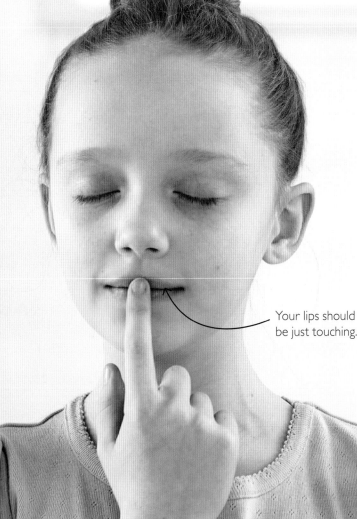

Your lips should be just touching.

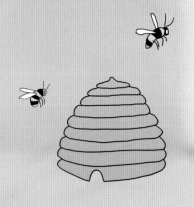

3

Rest your hands on your knees, sit up straight, and fill your body with a big breath. Close your eyes and see how long you can hum for using just one breath. Do this three more times.

4

Now, use your fingers to close your ears and take another big breath in through your nose. Make a bee sound again as you breathe out. Can you hear it inside your head?

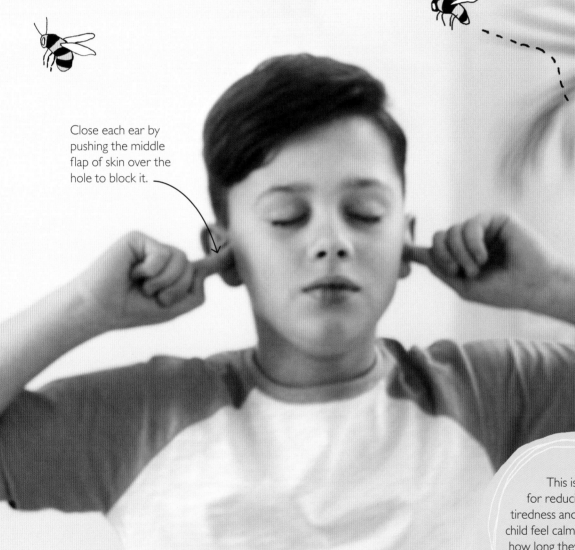

Close each ear by pushing the middle flap of skin over the hole to block it.

This is great for reducing mental tiredness and making your child feel calm. Silently count how long they can do it for and let them know how well they are doing.

FOR THE GROWN-UPS...

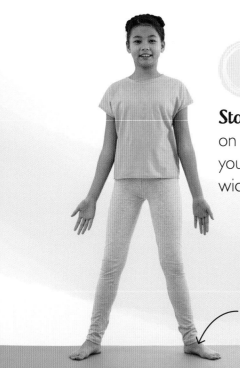

Start by standing on your mat with your feet slightly wider than your hips.

Point your toes slightly outward.

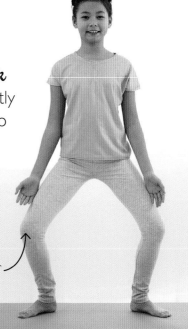

Keep your back straight and gently lower yourself into a squat position. Stop when your hips are lower than your knees.

Bend your knees.

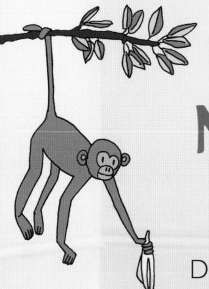

Monkey squat

Do you like monkeying around? Sink down into a squat and reach your arm up, just like a playful monkey.

Imagine you are hanging from a

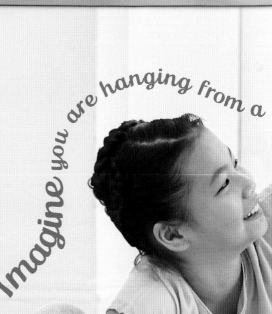

Keep your bottom off the floor.

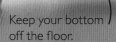

③

Bring your hands together into Namaste position.

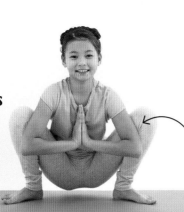

Push your arms into your legs.

Squatting is particularly good for strengthening the entire lower body. This pose is also thought to aid digestion.

FOR THE GROWN-UPS...

tree in the jungle.

Keep your knees back.

④

Reach down and rest your right hand on the floor. Raise your left hand into the air and look up toward it. Switch arms when you're ready.

Try this

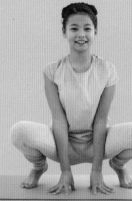

If you can't get your feet to the floor, try the frog squat. Putting your hands on the mat will stop you from feeling wobbly.

Reach up with your arms.

If you're a perfect primate, take your Monkey Squat one step further and raise both hands off the floor.

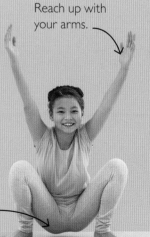

Don't let your bottom touch the floor.

55

Seated twist

This twist is fun to do and will make your back strong and flexible. It's important to do the pose in both directions. Imagine you are a fish twisting as you leap out of the water!

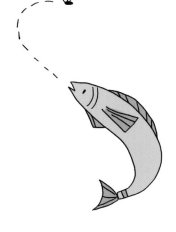

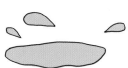

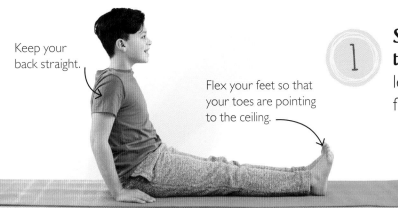

Keep your back straight.

Flex your feet so that your toes are pointing to the ceiling.

1 **Start by sitting on the floor** with your legs straight out in front of you.

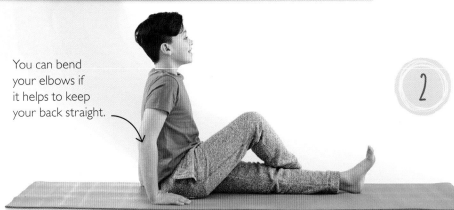

You can bend your elbows if it helps to keep your back straight.

2 **Bend your right leg,** then cross it over the left leg. Press your right foot into the floor.

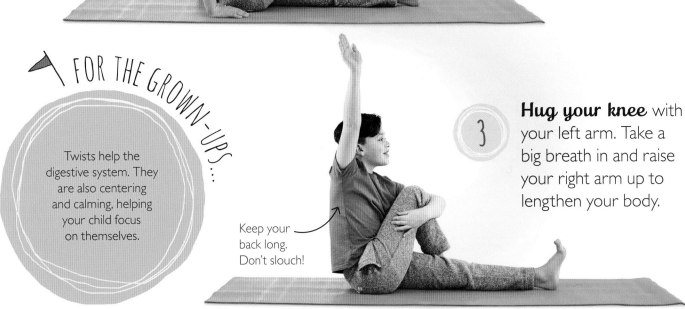

FOR THE GROWN-UPS...

Twists help the digestive system. They are also centering and calming, helping your child focus on themselves.

Keep your back long. Don't slouch!

3 **Hug your knee** with your left arm. Take a big breath in and raise your right arm up to lengthen your body.

Try this

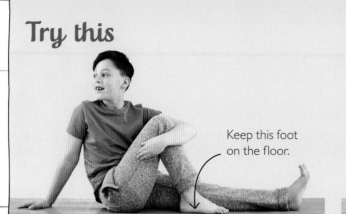

Keep this foot on the floor.

If the Seated Twist Pose is difficult, try this trick to make it easier: bend one leg up but keep your foot on the same side, then twist your body.

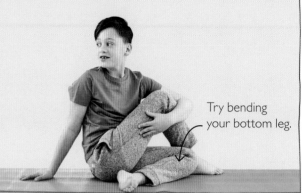

Try bending your bottom leg.

When you are comfortable in your Seated Twist, see if you can bend the bottom leg so that your foot is by your bottom.

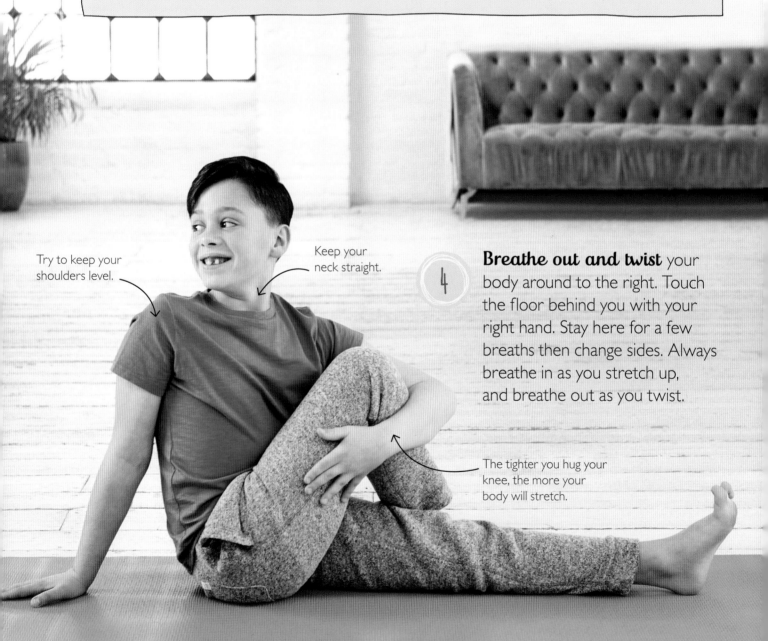

Try to keep your shoulders level.

Keep your neck straight.

4

Breathe out and twist your body around to the right. Touch the floor behind you with your right hand. Stay here for a few breaths then change sides. Always breathe in as you stretch up, and breathe out as you twist.

The tighter you hug your knee, the more your body will stretch.

Cow face

In this pose, the body is meant to look like a cow's face—your arms make a pair of cow ears and your legs become the cow's mouth. Let's see if you can make your body into this shape.

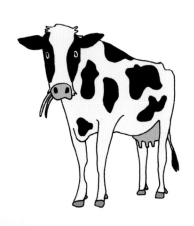

Keep your head and neck as straight as you can.

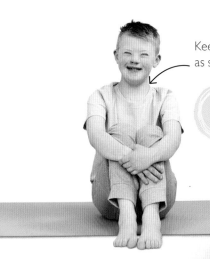

1 **Start by sitting down** with your knees bent and your feet on the floor.

2 **Slide your left foot** under the right leg, so that your left knee is on the floor in front of you and your left foot is next to your bottom.

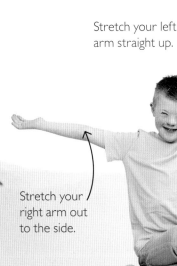

Your knees should be stacked on top of each other.

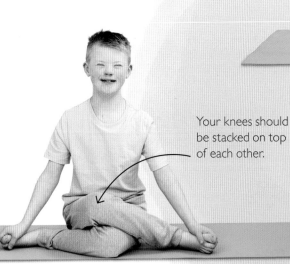

3 **Next lift your right leg** so that it crosses over the left and your right foot is next to your bottom.

Stretch your left arm straight up.

Stretch your right arm out to the side.

4 **Breathe in and stretch your left arm** straight up toward the ceiling and your right arm out to your right side.

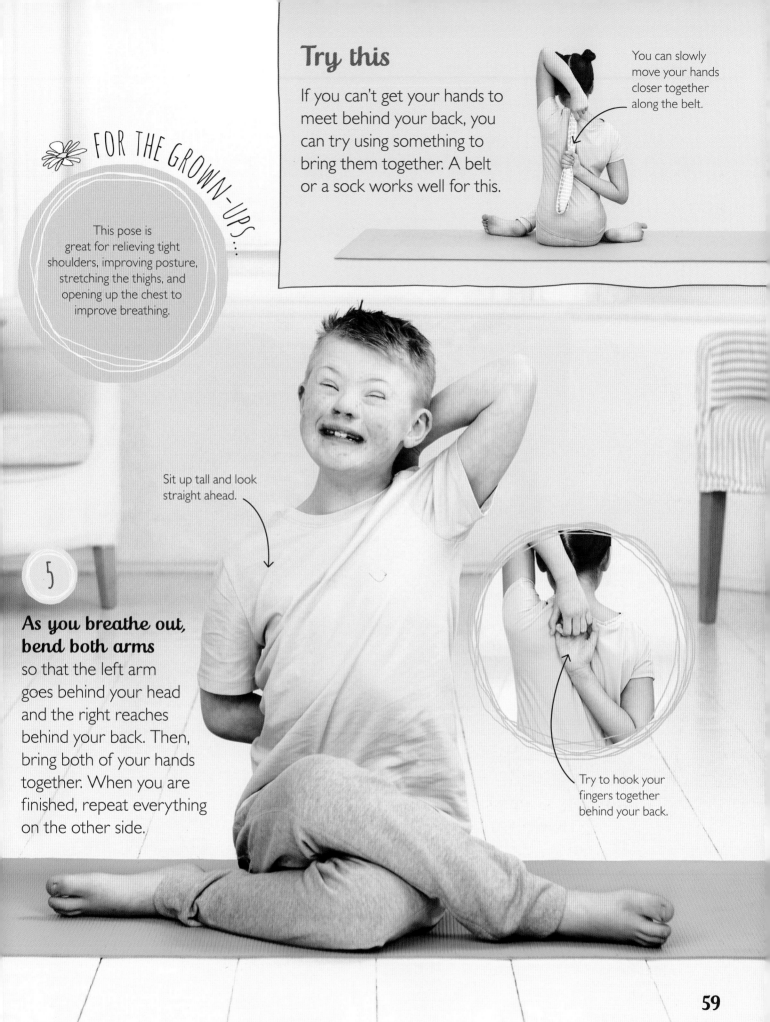

This pose is great for relieving tight shoulders, improving posture, stretching the thighs, and opening up the chest to improve breathing.

Try this

If you can't get your hands to meet behind your back, you can try using something to bring them together. A belt or a sock works well for this.

You can slowly move your hands closer together along the belt.

Sit up tall and look straight ahead.

5

As you breathe out, bend both arms so that the left arm goes behind your head and the right reaches behind your back. Then, bring both of your hands together. When you are finished, repeat everything on the other side.

Try to hook your fingers together behind your back.

Calming sequence

This sequence is perfect to do at night before you go to bed, or at any time when you need to calm down.

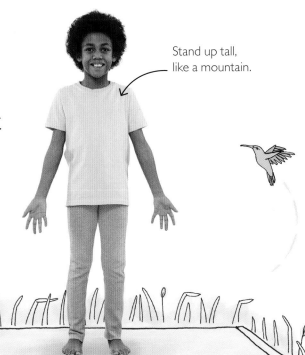

Stand up tall, like a mountain.

1 Mountain

Start by standing up straight in Mountain Pose, with your feet slightly apart. Breathe slowly through your nose.

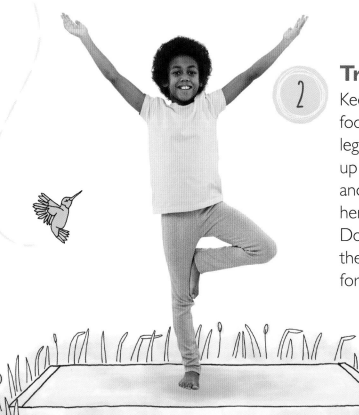

2 Tree

Keep one leg strong with the foot planted as you lift the other leg up to become a tree. Reach up to the sky with your branches and keep your head still. Stay here for five to ten breaths. Do the same on the other side, then go back to Mountain Pose for a few moments.

3

Standing Forward Bend

Stand straight, then slowly roll forward. Keep your legs bent to help you relax. Feel the weight of your head hanging down and touch the ground with your hands. Stay here for five to ten breaths. When you've finished, sit down on the floor.

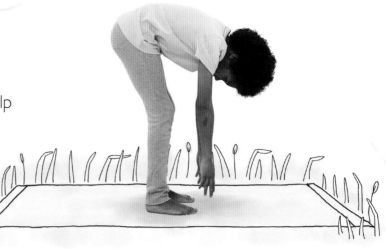

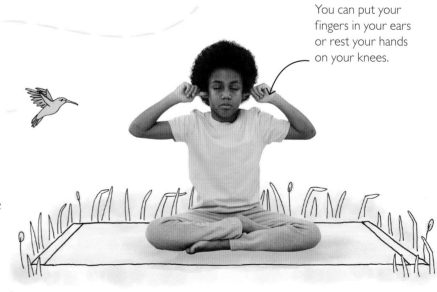

Bend one leg over the other.

4

Seated Twist

Turn into Seated Twist Pose and stay for a few breaths. Then breathe in and stretch up before breathing out and turning your body the other way into an Open Twist Pose. Repeat both twists with the other leg.

You can put your fingers in your ears or rest your hands on your knees.

5

Humming Bee

Sit back and practice your Humming Bee breath. Switch between making a bee noise and breathing normally. Do this three times. When you have finished your breathing exercises, slowly open your eyes.

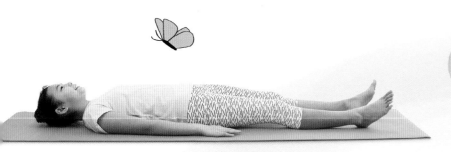

1 **Lie flat on your back** with your arms next to your body and your palms facing down.

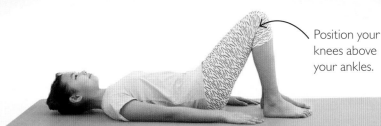

2 **Keeping your back and arms on the ground,** bend both knees. Keep your knees and feet hip-width apart, and your feet and all your toes on the floor.

Position your knees above your ankles.

This pose should make you feel full of energy!

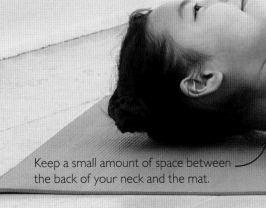

Keep a small amount of space between the back of your neck and the mat.

Keep your hands and arms flat on the floor.

Little bridge

Here's how to make your body into a bridge. The bridge should be just high enough to let a little stream run underneath it.

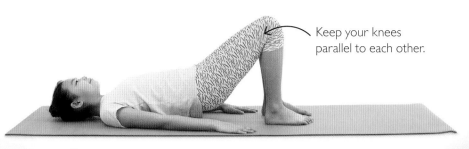

Keep your knees parallel to each other.

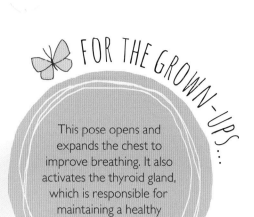

This pose opens and expands the chest to improve breathing. It also activates the thyroid gland, which is responsible for maintaining a healthy metabolism.

3 **Push your feet into the floor** and lift up your bottom and lower back off the ground.

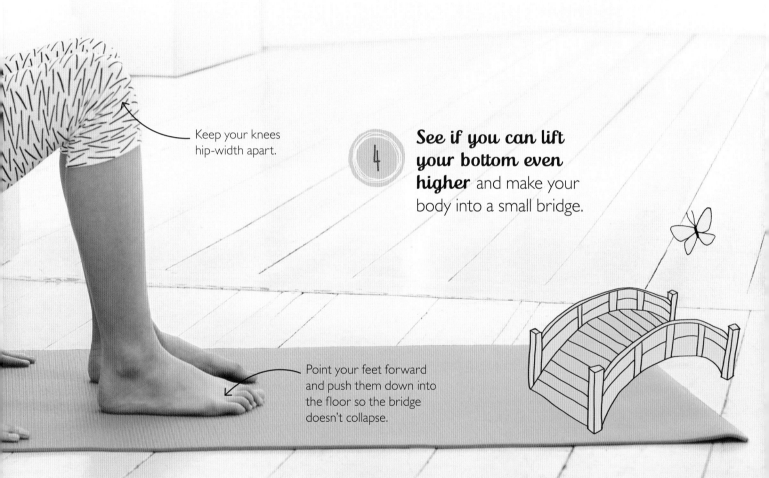

Keep your knees hip-width apart.

4 **See if you can lift your bottom even higher** and make your body into a small bridge.

Point your feet forward and push them down into the floor so the bridge doesn't collapse.

Try this

Once you're able to hold Bridge Pose, see if you can link your hands together underneath your lifted back.

Push the sides of your wrists into the floor to support you.

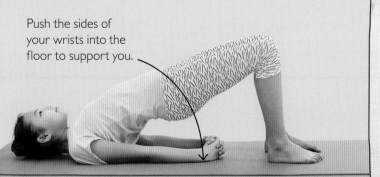

Half shoulder stand

Being upside down can make you feel great! Try it out with this fun pose that makes your tummy muscles stronger. You will need a pillow or a yoga block.

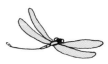

Lie on your back and hug your knees. Try to keep your back and shoulders relaxed.

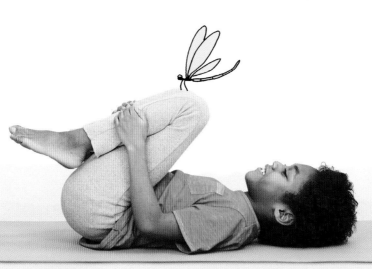

2

Put your arms by your sides and lift up your feet. See if you can put a pillow or a block on your feet—you might need someone else to do this part for you.

Keep the soles of your feet flat.

Stretch your arms down by your sides, with the palms of your hands on the mat.

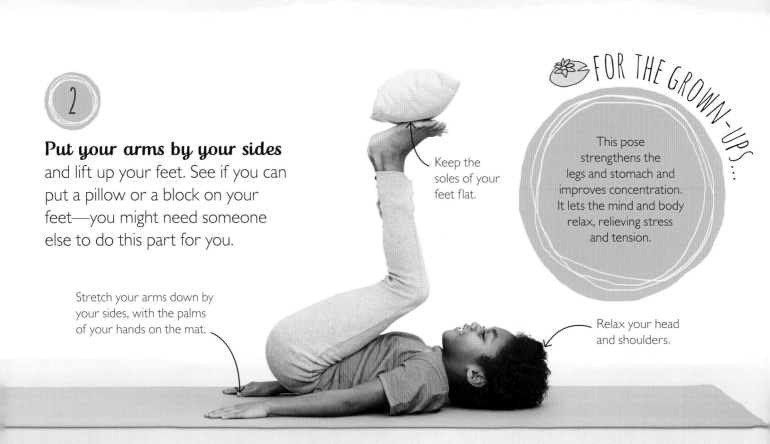

Relax your head and shoulders.

FOR THE GROWN-UPS...

This pose strengthens the legs and stomach and improves concentration. It lets the mind and body relax, relieving stress and tension.

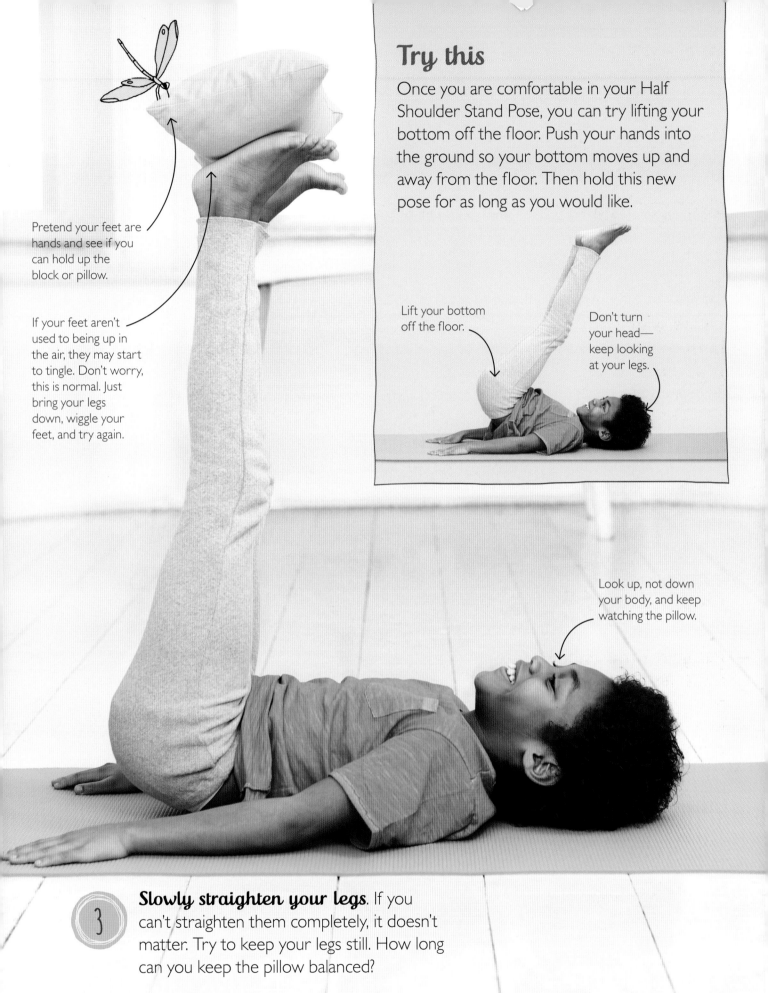

Pretend your feet are hands and see if you can hold up the block or pillow.

If your feet aren't used to being up in the air, they may start to tingle. Don't worry, this is normal. Just bring your legs down, wiggle your feet, and try again.

Try this

Once you are comfortable in your Half Shoulder Stand Pose, you can try lifting your bottom off the floor. Push your hands into the ground so your bottom moves up and away from the floor. Then hold this new pose for as long as you would like.

Lift your bottom off the floor.

Don't turn your head— keep looking at your legs.

Look up, not down your body, and keep watching the pillow.

3 **Slowly straighten your legs.** If you can't straighten them completely, it doesn't matter. Try to keep your legs still. How long can you keep the pillow balanced?

Restful
relaxation

It's really important to relax at the end of a yoga session, to allow the body and mind to rest. Anytime you want to unwind, you can lie down in Relaxation Pose.

When you **relax**, your body temperature drops. Make sure you are

FOR THE GROWN-UPS...

Asking kids to focus on their breathing will make their minds and bodies slow down. Relaxation after yoga allows the body to absorb all the benefits of the poses.

1

Lie on your back with your legs straight out in front of you. Place your arms by your sides with your palms facing upward. Close your eyes and relax.

2

Focus on your breathing. Allow your body to relax a little more each time you breathe out. Breathe in and out slowly and steadily through your nose.

3

You can stay in this pose for as long as you like. When you've finished, roll onto one side and sit up. Bring your hands together into Namaste position in front of your chest.

warm enough before you start, to keep yourself **comfortable.**

Think about how your tummy lifts when you breathe in and drops when you breathe out.

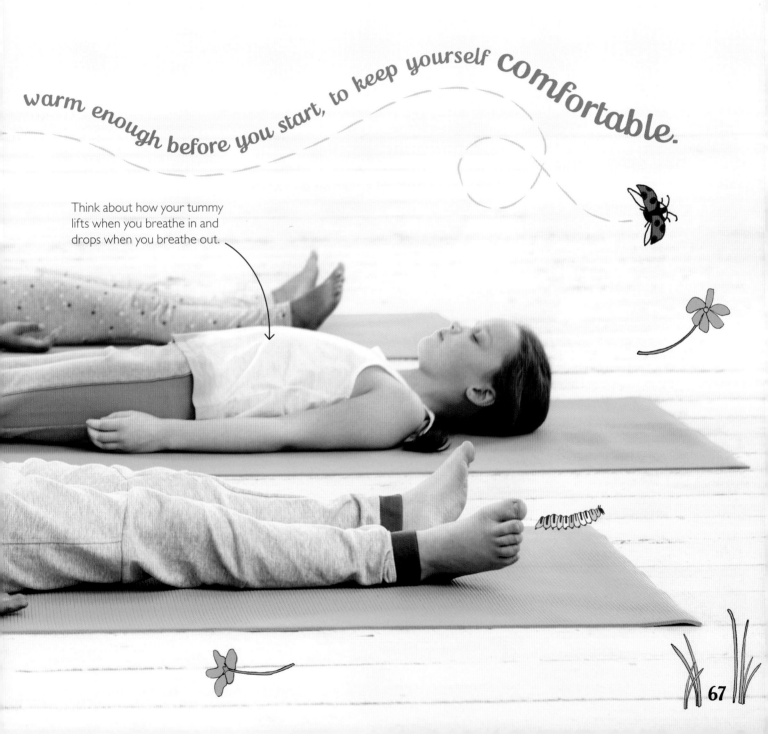

Parts of the body

To help you remember what the different parts of your body are called and where they're found, take a look at these three handy pictures.

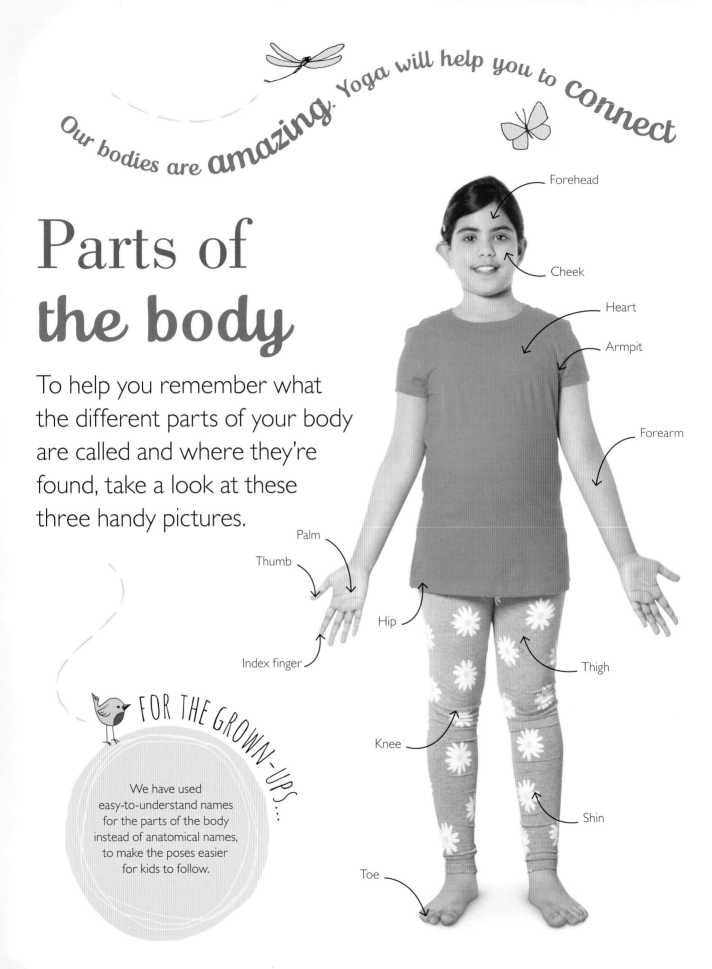

Forehead

Cheek

Heart

Armpit

Forearm

Palm

Thumb

Hip

Index finger

Thigh

Knee

Shin

Toe

FOR THE GROWN-UPS...

We have used easy-to-understand names for the parts of the body instead of anatomical names, to make the poses easier for kids to follow.

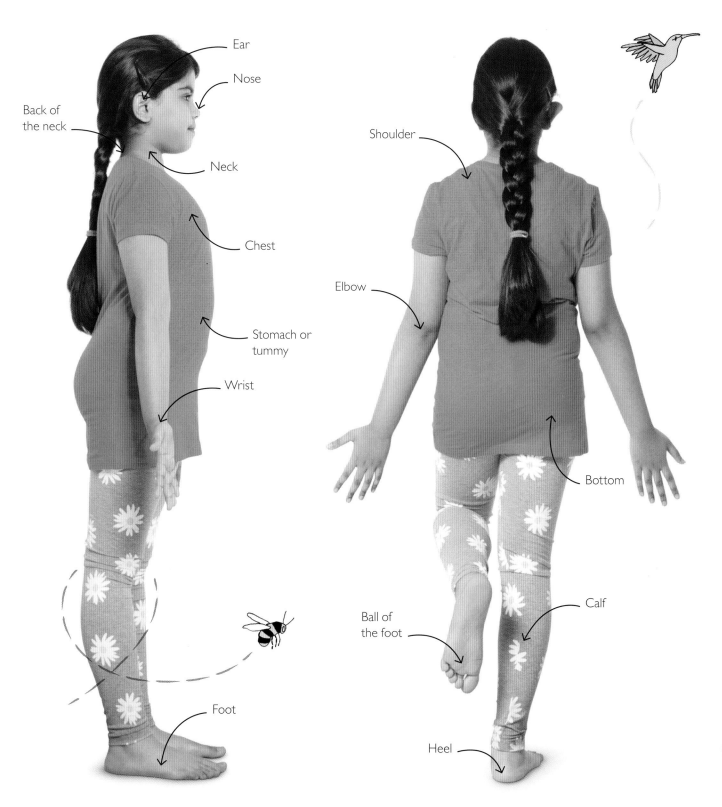

Ear

Nose

Back of the neck

Neck

Chest

Stomach or tummy

Wrist

Foot

Shoulder

Elbow

Bottom

Ball of the foot

Calf

Heel

Glossary

energizing
When something makes you feel full of energy

flex
Bend or move your muscles or a part of your body. If you are sitting on the floor and you flex your feet, they should be stretched upward, at right-angles to your legs.

hip-width
Distance between the outer edges of your feet, when you stand with your feet directly under your hips

massage
Squeeze or rub a part of the body to ease pain or relax someone

mindfulness
Awareness of your thoughts, emotions, and the world around you

namaste
[NAH-mah-stay]
Respectful way of greeting someone. It means "I see the best in you"

Om
The sound of the universe. When chanted by someone, it reminds them that we are all connected and it can help to focus the mind

parallel
When two things are the same distance apart along their whole length. If a stick is parallel to the floor, it is the same distance away at both ends and in the middle

pose
A particular way of holding your body or sitting, standing, or lying

relaxed
When you relax a part of your body, so it feels loose and less stiff

rotate
Turn in a circular movement

sequence
A number of things that are done one after the other in a certain order

stretch
Extend or lengthen something, for example, a muscle

tense
When you tense a muscle, you make it tight instead of relaxed

yoga
[YO-gah]
Sanskrit word meaning "union," which refers to the way that yoga connects the mind and body

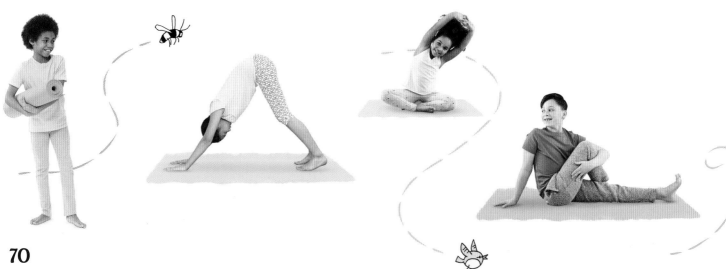

Sanskrit words

Yoga was created in India around 5,000 years ago by people who used a language called Sanskrit [SAN-skrit]. Most yoga poses have a Sanskrit name as well as an English name. Here is a list of some important yoga poses and their Sanskrit and English names.

Adho mukha Svanasana
[AD-ho MOO-ka SVAN-ah-sah-na]
Downward Dog Pose

Ananda Balasana
[an-NAN-dah BAL-ah-sah-na]
Happy Baby Pose

Ardha Matsyendrasana
[AR-da MAT-say-en-DRA-sah-na]
Seated Twist

Ardha Salamba sarvangasana
[AR-da sa-LAM-ba SAR-vang-gah-sah-na]
Half Shoulder Stand

Asana
[AH-sah-na]
Pose or posture. Most yoga positions will have a name that ends in this word.

Balasana
[bal-AH-sah-na]
Child's Pose

Brahmari
[bra-MAR-ree]
Humming Bee

Bhujangasana
[boo-jang-GAH-sah-na]
Cobra Pose

Dhanurasana
[DAN-ur-ar-SAH-na]
Bow Pose

Garudasana
[ga-roo-DA-sah-na]
Eagle Pose

Gomukhasana
[go-MOOK-ah-sah-na]
Cow Face Pose

Hindolasana
[hin-DOE-la-sah-na]
Rock the Baby

Malasana
[ma-LA-sah-na]
Squat

Marjariasana
[mar-JAR-ee-ah-SAH-na]
Cat Pose

Navasana
[NA-vah-SAH-na]
Boat Pose

Setu Bandha Sarvangasana
[SET-oo BAND-ah sar-van-GAH-sah-na]
Bridge Pose

Simhasana
[SIM-ha-sah-na]
Lion Pose

Tadasana
[TAD-AH-sah-na]
Mountain Pose

Utkatasana
[OOT-KAT-AH-sah-na]
Chair Pose

Uttanasana
[OO-tan-AH-sah-na]
Standing Forward Bend

Virabhadrasana I
[vir-ra-bha-DRA-sah-na I]
Warrior I Pose

Virabhadrasana II
[vir-ra-bha-DRA-sah-na 2]
Warrior II Pose

Vrksasana
[VRIK-sha-sah-na]
Tree Pose

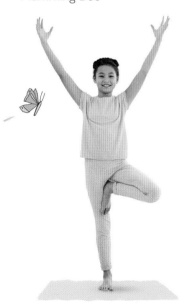
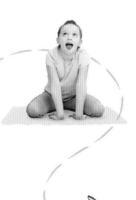
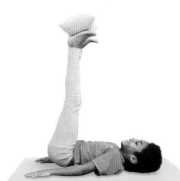
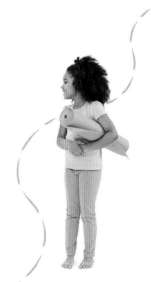

Index

A

arm stretches 27

B

back stretches 14–15, 20–21, 27
balance 28–29, 36–37, 40–41, 46–47
Boat Pose 28–29, 45
bones 12, 48
Bow Pose 22–23, 31
brain 18, 52
breathing 8–9, 20, 26–27, 59, 63, 66–67
breathing exercises 52–53
Bridge Pose 62–63

C

calmness 8, 53, 56, 60–61
Cat-Cow Pose 14–15, 17
Chair Pose 38–39, 45
chanting 9
chest 20, 59, 63
Child's Pose 26–27
Cobra Pose 20–21, 30
concentration 64
confidence sequence 44–45
Cow Face Pose 58–59
cushions 64, 65

D

Downward Dog 18–19, 30

E

Eagle Pose 40–41, 45
energy 18, 30–31, 36, 41, 62
Extended Puppy Pose 19

F

flexibility 15, 20
focus 8, 36, 56
Frog Squat 55
full body stretches 40–41

G

growth spurts 12, 48

H

Half Shoulder Stand 64–65
hamstrings 12
Happy Baby Pose 50–51
Humming Bee Breath 52–53, 61

L

leg strengthening 6, 38–39
leg stretches 13, 17, 34–35, 49
Lion Pose 24–25, 31
Low Lunge 34–35

M

mental relaxation 33, 64, 66
mental tiredness 52, 53
Monkey Squat 54–55
Mountain Pose 32–33, 41, 44, 60
muscle tightness 12, 48

N

Namaste 8–9, 31, 33, 67
neck tension 15

O, P

Om 9
Peaceful Warrior Pose 43
posture 33, 38, 59

R

Relaxation Pose 66–67
rocking the baby 12–13, 17

S

Seated Side Stretch 11, 16
Seated Twist 56–57, 61
shoulder stands 64–65
shoulder stretches 10–11, 16, 27
shoulder tension 15, 59
shrugs 10, 16

side stretches 11, 16, 46

Sphinx Pose 21
spine 15, 18, 20, 23
squatting 54–55
stability 36
Standing Forward Bend 48–49, 61
stomach 64
strength 33, 36–37, 42–43, 44
stress 64
Surfer 43
Swaying Palm Tree Pose 46

T

Table Pose 14, 30
thigh muscles 38, 59
Three-Legged Dog Pose 19
Tiger Pose 15
tongue 24–25
Tree Pose 46–47, 60
tummy muscles 28, 29, 34, 35, 64
twists 56–57

W

warm-up sequence 16–17
Warrior I Pose 36–37
Warrior II Pose 42–43, 44

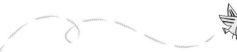

Acknowledgments

DK would like to thank the following: Alfie, Ava, Brooke, Calum, Ishani, Kayleb, and Lindsay for modeling; model agencies Zebedee Management and Urban Angels; Claire Henshaw for hair and make-up; Rachael Parfitt and Grace Poulter for styling; Steve Crozier for design help; Caroline Hunt for proofreading; Helen Peters for indexing; Sakshi Saluja for picture research.

The publisher would like to thank the following for their kind permission to reproduce their photographs:
(Key: a-above; b-below/bottom; c-center; f-far; l-left; r-right; t-top): **33 Dreamstime.com:** Ruzanna Arutyunyan (c).
68–69 Dorling Kindersley: Gaurav Chaudhary. **72 Dorling Kindersley:** Gaurav Chaudhary (br).

All other images © Dorling Kindersley
For further information see: www.dkimages.com

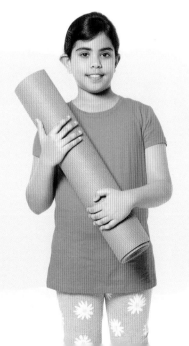